# New Hope for the Arthritic

BY THE SAME AUTHORS

*The Arthritic's Cookbook*

# New Hope
## for the Arthritic

Collin H. Dong, M.D.
and Jane Banks

**GRANADA**
London Toronto Sydney New York

Granada Publishing Limited
Frogmore, St Albans, Herts AL2 2NF
and
3 Upper James Street, London W1R 4BP
866 United Nations Plaza, New York, NY 10017, USA
117 York Street, Sydney, NSW 2000, Australia
100 Skyway Avenue, Rexdale, Ontario M9W 3A6, Canada
PO Box 84165, Greenside, 2034 Johannesburg, South Africa
CML Centre, Queen & Wyndham Streets, Auckland 1,
New Zealand

First published in Great Britain by
Hart-Davis, MacGibbon Ltd 1976
Reissued by Granada Publishing 1980

ISBN 0 246 10951 3

Printed in Great Britain by
Richard Clay (The Chaucer Press) Ltd.,
Bungay, Suffolk

Granada ®
Granada Publishing ®

*This book is dedicated to the following Dongs:*

Ten-Song (Guiding Star) Dong, my father
Yuk-Gee (Jade Pearl) Dong, my mother
Mil-lie (Elegant Beauty) Dong, my wife

# Acknowledgements

I would like to express my gratitude and thanks to the following persons:

To Jane Banks, my co-author, who insisted that we simply must write a second book to answer the many enquiries prompted by the first book. Although my work as a doctor and businessman kept me busy from 8 A.M. to 7 P.M. daily, I was sure that I could cut down on a few hours of sleep to write the book. Having been convinced that it was important to explain my theory, I agreed to write the text of the book and to have Mrs Banks do the recipes.

To Cynthia Vartan, my editor at Thomas Y. Crowell Company, who sent back my first draft, saying that all it needed was organisation. Her confidence that I could write the book gave me the impetus to continue working on it.

To Dr S. I. Hayakawa, my friend, who read the first draft and gave me invaluable suggestions about organising it.

To Galen, my son, who planned my twenty-four-hour day so that I could find at least four hours a day to work on this book. He even gave me six hours on Wednesdays to play golf.

To Eileen and Colleen, my daughters, for their time, their research and their work in taking dictation and in transcription and revision of my copy.

And last, but certainly not least, to Mil-lie, my wife, who tolerated my changes in mood, temper and ideas. She sat for over twelve months taking dictation on thousands of pages of paper and then taking dictation on the revisions of each page. Her talent and skill as a typist saw me through this ordeal. Her capacity for work, judgement and organisation were intrinsic to the completion of this book. But most of all, I am grateful for her love and affection.

# Contents

# RECIPES

# Introduction

This book is based, first of all, on my own experience of having and recovering from a severe form of arthritis. It is further based on thirty-seven years of using my own dietary therapy on patients suffering from the same or similar ailments. It is not a scientific work, in the sense of being based on thorough and well-authenticated scientific research.

What worked for me has achieved remarkable results for thousands of my patients. Many, in turn, referred to me other sufferers from arthritis – and they too found relief from their pains after following my regimen.

I would have started shouting from the housetops that I had made a great medical discovery, except for the following facts. First, when I made the initial discovery of my method, I was a young doctor, and by no means ready to challenge medical orthodoxy. Second, I felt that I needed more experience.

The orthodox view on the subject of arthritis is dogmatic – and who was I to question the distinguished group of organised doctors who constitute the American Arthritis Foundation? In a booklet entitled *Arthritis – the Basic Facts* they said:

'People insist on believing that special diets or exotic foods are helpful in arthritis.

'The possible relationship of diet and arthritis has been thoroughly and scientifically studied.

'The simple proven fact is: no food has anything to do with causing arthritis and no food is effective in treating or "curing" it.

'The proper diet for someone with arthritis is a normal,

well-balanced, nourishing diet – the same things people
without arthritis should eat.'

Those were pretty intimidating words! Here I was, beginning to believe, because of my own experience, that there
*was* a connection between diet and arthritis. And there was
the learned foundation announcing, as if with the voice of
Jehovah: '*The relationship between diet and arthritis has been
thoroughly and scientifically studied. The simple proven fact
is: no food has anything to do with causing arthritis and no
food is effective in treating or "curing" it.*'

Those formidable words sound final. Yet I could not
accept their finality.

What is the state of the medical art so far as arthritis is
concerned? Medical scientists all over the world – bio-
chemists, immunologists, researchers conducting experiments on animals, others using sophisticated modern
instruments of analysis – are trying, without success, to find
the cause and cure of this dreaded disease.

Fifty million people in the United States and five million
in Great Britain suffer from arthritis at one or another level
of severity – so the reader certainly either has it himself or is
related to someone who has. Arthritis afflicts children as
well as centenarians. And all those afflicted are in pain; in
America 400 million dollars is spent annually on ineffective
'cures' and over-the-counter pain-killers.

The orthodox treatment everywhere is large doses of
aspirin. Proprietary drugs, developed as substitutes for
aspirin, are also used – and some are selling like hot cakes.
But all these drugs treat the symptoms, not the disease.

Consequently, once a diagnosis of arthritis is made, most
patients are told in effect: 'There is no cure for your ailment.
You will simply have to live with it.' They face years of
recurrent, persistent, irritating pain and disability – wishing
desperately for something, anything, to do about it!

When I was thirty-five years old, only seven years out of
Stanford Medical School and my subsequent internship at
San Francisco General Hospital, I was afflicted with arthritis.
As it steadily became worse, with crippling pain in my joints,
I also developed a severe generalised dermatitis.

I searched through my medical textbooks, through other books, and journals. I consulted my former professors and my medical colleagues. In three long years of progressively increasing suffering I found that there was nothing that doctors could do for me except to prescribe large doses of aspirin – which was precisely what was giving me my skin disorder. I was genuinely at a dead end, doomed, as far as I could see, to unrelieved misery for the rest of my days.

When I recently told this story to my friend Dr S. I. Hayakawa, the eminent semanticist and educator, he was reminded of a motto of his mentor, Count Alfred Korzybski, the founder of General Semantics: 'When things are really hopeless, that is where hope begins.' In my preoccupation with acquiring a Western scientific education and becoming a physician in the Western sense, I had forgotten my background in Chinese culture. In my illness I became desperate enough to be thrown back to it. As I explain later in this book, I devised a simplified Chinese diet based on the simple food of my childhood – mainly fish, chicken, vegetables and rice.

Two years ago I collaborated with my friend and former patient Mrs Jane Banks in writing *The Arthritic's Cookbook*, a book of recipes using the foods allowed on my diet. Mrs Banks, a talented cook and experienced hostess, had been a victim of severe and crippling arthritis.

As a result of that book we received thousands of letters from readers all over the United States, Canada and parts of Europe. Many of the letters substantiated my hypothesis. Many of them, moreover, stimulated further questions about the diet and about various aspects of arthritis, and raised other enquiries which this book attempts to answer.

The present volume, then, has four purposes:

First, to give more information on rheumatic diseases so that the patient will have a clearer understanding of the illness, its course and its nature – making it possible for him to cooperate with his own doctor.

Second, to give an explanation of my dietary regimen, not only for arthritis sufferers but also for my medical colleagues, so that they may use it as an auxiliary treatment for their rheumatic disease patients. Since the diet is intended as an adjunctive treatment, the arthritis victim can start on the diet plan at any time.

Third, to give more elaborate menus than were included in *The Arthritic's Cookbook* to make it easier to maintain the diet for longer periods of time, and to facilitate daily cooking and meal preparation by providing more recipes and cooking tips.

Finally, it is Mrs Banks's hope, and mine, that the reader may, with the help of this book, enjoy freedom from pain, and therefore a healthier, happier and longer life.

Several of my medical colleagues, knowing that I was working on this second book, sent statements expressly for publication endorsing my dietary precepts. I have chosen two of them for inclusion here.

The first is from Dr Ione E. Railton, who has been Associate Clinical Professor of Medicine at the University of California Medical School since 1947.

'I believe that excellent results really need a commendation. My sister Varian, whom Dr Dong has treated for the past year, has had such a remarkable turn-about in her health. She had an acute onset of rheumatoid arthritis at the age of fifty-five. The pain in her sternum and ribs was like angina, and we thought it was, until she was certain that it was related chiefly to the motions of deep breathing, turning over in bed and twisting. Next her hips became painful and she had difficulties rising from chairs. Then quite quickly came swollen, tender knees and ankles. She could barely walk and found the vibrations of car riding also caused pain. A rheumatologist put her on aspirin, cortisone and finally Indocid, which did help remarkably as long as she kept on a fairly high dosage regularly. She gained weight, her blood pressure became elevated and she was constantly fatigued and became desperately ill, to a point where she could not perform even the most menial task.

'She had heard of Dr Dong's successful treatment of arthritis with a dietary programme. So I arranged an appointment for her in March 1972. She felt better after her second visit. Wisely, Dr Dong took her off her medications very slowly – two months, I recall, to taper down the cortisone. He put her on an elimination diet.

'I had interned under Dr Albert Rowe, Sr, the eminent allergist, at the University of California, who published wheatless, milkless, eggless diets for hay fever, asthma and urticaria, and I reinforced the importance of diet to her. Besides, we come from an allergic family, both sides having pollen hay fever. She also exercised under warm water, slowly and to the point of relaxation, not muscle fatigue. I can state that she was a faithful adherent to Dr Dong's programme and added to her diet only on his advice, not on mine or her San Diego physician's. Every day she felt better. She lost forty pounds, and naturally looked younger, took over more housekeeping duties, socialised with her two daughters and grandchildren. She even went on car rides, a bus trip and this year, a trip to Canada.

'On our recent visit, she seemed entirely well except for easy fatiguability. No more ugly ankles, knee swellings and I think she could jitterbug with the same old zest – could she find one of us to keep up with her!

'In my clinic work, I've seen a lot of arthritis, rheumatoid and osteoarthritis. I was practising when cortisone was discovered in 1949. We used it in 1950 with marvellous results. Patients got better almost at once, they threw away their crutches and walked, the pain disappeared as well as did the swelling. We were all euphoric, patients and doctors; then came the side effects and our disillusionment: ulcers, hypertension, diabetes and moon faces. We had to quit our generous doses, use it only for handling acute episodes and again rely on aspirin, physiotherapy and supportive measures.

'Chronic diseases are always hard to handle, for they involve patients, family, employers and social services. I knew the future for my sister better than she – that we were all being involved in her health adjustment. Emotional factors play an important role in rheumatoid arthritis, so we all tried to alleviate her stress and anxiety. That is not easy in present everyday living. Now that we have a new approach to this problem which is geared to the total patient, his diet, his general health measures, exercise, acupuncture, I think rheumatoid arthritis will not be as devastating a problem as it was to all of us involved. But it takes interest on the part of the doctor in all facets of the disease and treatment, and a better-than-usual cooperation from the patient. That may mean frequent appointments, education, reassurance and modification of environment.

'Dr Dong has pointed the way, and his results are obvious. His patients are working and walking again!'

The second statement is from Dr John R. Upton, who graduated from the Stanford University School of Medicine in 1934. He was certified by the American Board of Obstetrics and Gynaecology and was the former chief of obstetrics and gynaecology at St Luke's Hospital, San Francisco. Dr Upton was also Associate Clinical Professor at the University of California Hospital, San Francisco.

'As a doctor of medicine, I have always been aware of the importance of a proper diet, and its full value was dramatically demonstrated through my personal experience this year. I was the victim of an arthritic condition which was increasingly painful. I had received the maximum amount of cortisone deemed advisable, and to resort to pain-killing drugs for the rest of my life was repugnant to me. It was then that I sought the help of Dr Collin Dong, whom I knew to be most successful in the treatment of this affliction.

'I am only one of Dr Dong's grateful patients who will be for ever indebted to him for his excellent care. To relieve my arthritic pains he outlined a plan which included a dietary regimen, moderate amounts of medication and exercise. The elimination of the overriding cause of the pain through a prescribed diet was a miracle.

'The delectable dietary regimen is fully outlined in Dr Dong's and Jane Banks's first book, *The Arthritic's Cookbook*, and it is the diet that I myself successfully followed.

'A cookbook is many things to many people. It can be a simple primer to initiate the aspiring novice. Again, it may present only the sophisticated dishes, tempting us by the richness of their sauces, the subtleties of their textures and flavour. For those who seek the exotic and unusual, there are books specialising in the cuisines of many lands, mysterious and foreign to our palate. Outranking all others is *The Arthritic's Cookbook*, which offers that treasure beyond measure, good health!

'Dr Dong's second book, *New Hope for the Arthritic*, furnishes a fuller explanation of his theories, including some of his clinical case histories. He includes his dietary regimen, and discusses the elimination of the ingredients which upset the body chemistry, causing pain and malfunction and resulting in physical incapacities. He also discusses proper nutrition.

'I hasten to point out that such a regimen does not deny one the joys of good food. As those who follow the suggested regimen in his books will discover, it offers a vast choice of nature's finest produce prepared with an endless variety of flavours, textures and seasonings.

'I recommend *New Hope for the Arthritic* to all who would find good fare, good health and the good life.'

I am deeply grateful to Drs Railton and Upton for their encouragement and support. It is good to know that their medical experience coincides so much with my own, especially on the question of the relation between diet, health *and illness*.

But I must come back to the fact mentioned at the beginning – that this book is the result of experience, and not of thoroughly tested and validated scientific theories. Such results on the subject of diet and illness are still to come.

I myself am not a research scientist. I am a practising doctor, immersed in the daily aches and pains and discomforts of a varied collection of patients of every race and nationality, from every walk of life. To discover the biochemical facts about the relation of diet to rheumatic diseases requires rigorous and painstaking research of a kind that I have neither the training nor the time to perform.

It is my sincere hope, therefore, that not only will sufferers from arthritis and rheumatic diseases be helped by this book, but also scientific investigators in this field will be stimulated by what I have written here to do more intensive research into the relationship between diet and arthritis.

# 1

## Diet and nutrition: an important but neglected subject

CASE HISTORY

NAME: Mr G. I.
RESIDENCE: California
AGE: 43
OCCUPATION: Manager of service bureau
DIAGNOSIS: Polyarthritis
DURATION: Five years
FIRST VISIT: 13 April 1973
PREVIOUS MEDICATION: Aspirin, Indocid, Butazolidin,
    Empirin (aspirin and caffeine) compound with codeine,
    Darvon, (propoxyphene), corticosteroid
INTERVIEWED: 26 January 1974

'The onset of my arthritis started about five years ago. It began in my right wrist, went down into my hip and also affected my sternum. My arthritis got worse and worse and I became more and more restricted and restrained. It was very frustrating to me.

'I went to several doctors and had different kinds of diagnoses. One doctor said it was early osteoarthritis. Another specialist said it was polyarthritis. They gave me various kinds of pain-killing medicines, but did not help me at all. So I finally went to the Rheumatic and Arthritis Disease Clinic in my home town. I was treated there for a year and a half. I was going through test after test until I felt like a human guinea pig. Because of my pain, they started giving me five different prescription drugs. They also gave me cortisone orally and by injection, and other types of pain-killers. All this was still doing me no good. You have no idea how desperate I began to get.

'I had to do a lot of sitting, walking, and sometimes running, in my job. I had also been very active in my personal life. I was an active member of the YMCA Youth Programme. We hike, camp and have many sports activities. Since the onset of my sickness, I could hardly carry on my job, and I had to give up participation in the YMCA for two years.

'I first saw Dr Dong on 13 April 1973.

[*Mr G. I.'s experience is typical of the manner in which some doctors treat rheumatic disease cases. Large doses of medication such as aspirin, Indocid, Butazolidin, codeine, Darvon, steroids and other medication are prescribed in desperation because the patient does not respond to their therapy programme. The fact that some patients might be allergic to any one of these drugs, thereby exacerbating the illness, is completely ignored.*

*When Mr G. I. came to my office, I analysed the previous treatment and suspected that he could be allergic to one of the chemicals in the medication that had been prescribed. The patient was advised to discontinue the medication except for Darvon, codeine and steroids for pain. He was given my usual lecture on the relation of nutrition to health and told to adhere strictly to the Dong Diet. He was given acupuncture treatments once a month.*

*On 26 January 1974, after eight months of treatment, the patient was practically rejuvenated. He had lost twenty-two pounds. His blood pressure, which was elevated before he came to my office, was normal. The patient no longer required any medication. His joint mobility was almost normal.*]

'Now I am a new man. A lot of things happened to me. My pain was alleviated almost immediately. I began to sleep better at night, and the anxiety that I had about all my problems began to go away. That diet is really something. I feel, as the Spanish say, "Muy macho". I feel that I am not limited at all now, or restrained in any of my activities. I feel ten or fifteen years younger, I can participate in the family sports and it is great. You do not realise what pain is, or was, until you get rid of it. I went back to my YMCA work and recently we went on a week-end overnight. We went on a fifteen mile hike down through the mountains and trails. I was able to climb like a young mountain goat.'

The great physician Sir William Osler once said, 'When I see an arthritic patient walk in the front door of my office, I want to walk out the back door.' In my office in San Francisco I have no back door. When new arthritic patients come painfully in or are helped in by their relatives, I have to accept the challenge they present to me. Every one of these patients is, like Mr G. I., a chronic case who has been treated by several doctors and clinics with orthodox methods. My office is a 'port of last resort'.

During the past thirty years I have read most of the periodicals, medical journals, books and scientific papers on rheumatic diseases. Whenever possible I attend clinical demonstrations and seminars throughout the world.

My own treatment for the arthritic patients who come to me is principally a dietary therapy, based on my belief that the causes of rheumatic diseases are chemical poisoning from the additives and preservatives that are put into our foods and from allergy to certain foods. In subsequent chapters I will go into my reasons for this theory in detail. I will also discuss the types of arthritis, their treatment by orthodox methods and my own treatment, longevity and exercise as they relate to the arthritic, and acupuncture as an adjunct to my treatment of the disease. I want to begin, however, with the all-important but neglected topics of diet and nutrition and how they affect our health and well-being, for an understanding of this is basic to everything else I will say.

Diet refers to the food that people eat while nutrition refers to the assimilation of food into the bloodstream so that it can be used by the human body. Perhaps the clearest way to show how the food we eat alters our whole body chemistry is first to give you a brief refresher course on the process of digestion.

When a housewife shops for the family meal, she usually brings home three basic materials: meat (including fats), vegetables and bread (carbohydrates). Most recipes are made from one or more of these three ingredients.

After you put the food into your mouth and start chewing it, digestion begins. The salivary gland enzymes begin changing the starch into maltose, and the food then passes down the oesophagus to the stomach, which is a food reservoir. The gastric juices, consisting mainly of hydrochloric acid, start mixing with the food. They also activate another enzyme called pepsin, which starts the protein digestion. As more food comes down into the stomach, the gastric muscles contract and mix the food thoroughly with the digestive juices. Soon it becomes a thick gruel, and gradually this gruel works down into the duodenum, which comprises the first twelve inches of the small intestine. It takes about four hours for the average meal to go through the stomach into the duodenum. There, other secretions, bile from the liver and alkaline pancreatic juice from the pancreas, neutralise the acid gruel. The function of the bile is to produce an alkaline reaction in the intestines, and the emulsification and absorption of fats.

The whole intestinal tract is twenty-six feet long. The upper part is the one-foot-long duodenum. The next part is called the jejunum, which is eight feet long and about one and a half inches in diameter. Then come the twelve feet of the slightly narrower ileum. The end of the ileum connects with the five-foot-long large intestine, in the right lower abdomen near your appendix.

To a large degree the upper intestines are free of microbes because stomach acid kills most of them. However, the lower intestines contain upwards of fifty varieties of bacteria, some which help in the digestion process.

When the gruel reaches the duodenum, it causes the duodenum to produce a hormone called secretin. Secretin goes through the blood to stimulate the pancreas into instant secretion of its alkaline digestive juices. Then these pour into the duodenum, neutralising the acids. The pancreatic juices also contain three important enzymes that break up the protein, fats and carbohydrates into basic building materials for the body. One of these enzymes, trypsin, initiates the breakdown of proteins into amino acids. Another, amylase, converts starches into carbohydrates in the form of glucose, and a third, lipase, attacks the fat globules, breaking them into fatty acids and glycerin. As these nutrients pass through the twenty-one feet of small intestines, the processed meal is absorbed into the bloodstream by millions of villimicroscopic, fingerlike projections on the walls of the intestines. The function of the villi is of the utmost importance. They separate the amino acids, glucose and fats from the waste material. The fats are absorbed and sent through the lymphatic vessels and then into the bloodstream. The amino acids and glucose are absorbed through capillaries of the villi and then into the liver. The processing of a meal usually takes from three to eight hours. The rest of the watery gruel goes into the large intestine. There the water is taken back into the bloodstream. Waste matter, including fibres and cellulose, are passed from the body as faecal matter.

After the digested meal has been absorbed through the millions of villi into the bloodstream, it goes through the liver, which is the great detoxifier. This means that the liver has the ability to change poisonous substances into non-poisonous chemicals. For instance, the steak that becomes amino acids in the intestines before it is absorbed into the bloodstream, cannot be used until the liver changes its character so that it is fit for human use, or else it would be poisonous. From the liver the processed meal goes with the returning bloodstream into the right side of the heart, then into the lungs, where the blood is refreshed by giving up carbon dioxide and absorbing oxygen. The refreshed blood with all its components is then returned to the left side of the heart, where it is pumped into the entire vascular system of 60,000 miles of blood vessels. The sixty trillion cells in the body of every human adult are supplied with oxygen and food by this process. (I will tell you more about this in the next chapter.)

All of the above discussion is a very sketchy description of

what happens to a meal. Actually the process is so complicated that scientists are constantly discovering new enzymes
and hormones that aid in the digestive process. The functioning of the human body in its entirety is a mystery that may
never be completely unravelled.

The groceries that were made into the evening meal have
now been mixed with the chemicals of the blood to become
part of the huge chemical plant in the body. There are
millions of chemical reactions taking place every second of
the day. In short, the foods that we consume give us the
energy and the basis of life. They perform this function
through the mechanical and chemical actions of the digestive
system and the trillions of cells in our body.

It should be fairly obvious by now that the quality and
quantity of food that we eat can and do alter the whole body
chemistry. The physiology and biochemistry of the body,
and the process of digestion have not changed much since
the time of Pleistocene man, approximately five hundred
thousand years ago. The present-day human being was
formed by the diet of the first man. There have been no
significant changes in the basic foodstuffs – meat, vegetables,
dairy products and carbohydrates (e.g. bread).

Industrialisation has given us many spectacular time-
saving conveniences. But when we include food processing
as a mark of achievement, with its addition of tons of
chemicals to colour food, to enhance its taste and to preserve
it, we have ignored what these added substances do to our
bodies. It is very likely that these added chemicals cause many
of the physical and mental disorders in our society today.

## A trip to Fantasyland

I recently asked fifty people – lawyers, accountants, insurance brokers, bankers and other non-medical people – what
is meant by the cellular structure of the human body. Not
one of them knew. Becoming better acquainted with the
marvellous structure of the human body and its functions is
not only a source of intellectual delight and satisfaction, but
it also gives one an approach to proper living. In order to

make this discussion clearer and more easily understood, I'm going to take you on a short trip to Fantasyland.

I live in San Francisco on top of the famous and historic Telegraph Hill. The view from my apartment gives a panoramic scene of the two bridges and the beautiful bay. One day recently, redevelopment started at the foot of Telegraph Hill. Demolition began on a large seventy-five-year-old cold-storage building. Instead of using the conventional steel ball to knock down the walls of the building, teams of workmen began taking it down brick by brick, perhaps because old bricks are more valuable today then newly manufactured ones.

This unusually slow method of disassembling a structure in these days of speed somehow excited my imagination. That night in my dreams, I found myself walking into the huge brick building at the foot of the hill. When I entered, I discovered an amazing interior. Not only were the walls made of bricks of all shapes, sizes and colours, but everything inside the building was also made of bricks. I ascended the stairway to the top floor where I saw a huge sculpture of a human head, complete in every detail – with brains, nerves, eyes, ears, nose, throat, mouth and neck. It was a beautiful mosaic – composed entirely of bricks. Walking down a spiral staircase built around the sculpture, I saw on the next floor an extension of this sculpture, a chest with lungs, heart, glands and all the blood vessels. This also was made in the same strange way – with bricks.

The next floor contained more of the sculpture – a replica of the abdomen, with the diaphragm, duodenum, small intestines, large intestines, liver, pancreas, kidneys and spleen. On the next floor were the reproductive organs of the female, the uterus, the tubes, the ovaries and also the bladder. Down again to another floor, and there was the reproductive system of the male with the genital organs. From the second floor down to the basement, the sculpture was of the two legs and feet, showing the muscular and bone structures of the limbs. To my surprise, on closer examination I found each one of these bricks was alive, and each was nourished by tiny vessels made of bricks.

Suddenly I was awakened by a telephone call. It was an unimportant call, but what was important was that I now had an idea of a novel way to present the human anatomy and physiology to my readers. For, to understand any medical subject, one must have some knowledge of the functions of the human body.

## *New concepts of microscopic anatomy and physiology*

The human body in its entirety is made up of about sixty trillion bricks, or cells, just like the sculpture in my Fantasyland. From here on, I will refer to the body cells as bricks because I think this is more picturesque and, I hope, easier for the reader to visualise.

The most wonderful process of life is the fertilisation of the egg brick by the sperm brick in the female body. At that moment the fertilised germ brick is a human individual in a one-brick stage of development. This brick then splits into two bricks and divides over and over again until a baby is formed. This process is similar to the construction of a building. The first brick must be laid, then many other bricks must be added in order to complete the building.

Early in their development, the bricks all look alike. But when more and more bricks are being reproduced, some begin to take on special characteristics and look different from the others. This is called the differentiation stage. Thus we have groups called muscle bricks, skin bricks, nerve bricks, connective tissue bricks and blood bricks.

Not only do they look different, they also have different purposes. The muscle bricks specialise in movement, the nerve bricks receive and transmit stimuli, epithelial bricks specialise in transporting oxygen and nutrients to all the other trillions of bricks, and connective tissue bricks form many structures of the body and hold all the parts together.

Each and every brick carries on all the processes of life – they live and die, they take in food, they eliminate waste, they respond to stimuli, they move, and they reproduce other bricks of their own kind. Of all the wonderful skills that the body is capable of performing, the unsurpassed accomplishment is its capacity to reproduce its own kind and pass on genetic substances for future generations.

Millions of bricks die every second, and just as many new ones are born. Skin bricks reproduce every ten to twelve hours; others, such as muscle and fat bricks, reproduce more slowly. Some bricks live longer than others. The only kinds that do not reproduce themselves are the brain bricks. Since you are supplied with more brain bricks than you will ever need in a lifetime, reproduction of these is not necessary. Also, nature seems to have made brain bricks stronger than most of the other trillions of bricks in the body because man's mental processes are still stable when many other groups of bricks are no longer functioning.

It is important to realise that each group of bricks in the human body is related to every other group. They somehow communicate with each other, possibly through enzymes or hormones, as well as through the nervous system.

When a person thinks, not only are the brain bricks used, but all the bricks in the body play some part in the thinking process. The muscle, the gland and the blood bricks, and even the bricks in the digestive system all team together as a unit to help in the function of thinking. If you walk, you do not walk with your legs alone; the brain bricks start out by giving you an idea, and all the other bricks in the whole system help you to arrive at your destination. Many other emotions, too, such as fear, hunger and other bodily states, require the action of the whole organism.

## Amazing new view of bricks (cells)

Recent basic research has brought to light a new concept of the functions of the sixty trillion bricks of our body. Very few people, including scientists, know that bricks have appetites and special diets. When I studied medicine, and up to a short time ago, the bricks of our body were considered just sacks containing fluid with chemicals and genetic substances. Research has given the bricks new and intricate characteristics. They live and die, they take in foods, they eliminate waste, they respond to stimuli, they move and reproduce their own kind.

A Nobel prize-winning scientist Dr Christian de Duve, Professor of Medicine at Rockefeller University, New York, suggested studying the diets of cancer cells, then slipping potent anti-cancer drugs into the food they liked best, and thus destroy them.

This book does not deal with cancer, although I mention it several times, and in order to explain this theory, it is enough to think of cancer cells as *criminals* in our orderly society. They are bricks that do not conform to orderly multiplications, they start multiplying without inhibition, thus causing growth, such as tumours. Tumours, because of their constant growth, cause neighbouring bricks to be crowded and injured, leading to malfunction. The cancer bricks can also spread through the bloodstream, causing tumours elsewhere in our body.

'Some cells in the human body are very avid eaters, others are less greedy. What is needed now,' says Dr de Duve, 'is a detailed inventory of the tastes of cells, and their favourite foodstuff.'

Dr de Duve and his group in Europe and the United States have been tying powerful anti-cancer drugs to a carrier. The goal would be to kill the cancer bricks without harming the good ones, should the appetites of the cancer bricks be found to be different. One need only think of putting poison on cheese for rats. This ties in quite well with my new concept of histology and physiology, and is the reason that I introduced, at this point, the subject of cancer, which vitally concerns everyone.

### Why does a person get sick?

How does all this relate to diet, nutrition, health and well-being? Well, each group of bricks has different functions, and therefore will require different types of nutrients. One group may want certain minerals, others may want some vitamins, glucose, and amino acids, and still others may want hormones. It all depends on the needs of each brick or group of bricks.

Let me give you a typical example of why someone gets sick. If before an evening meal John Jones drinks three or more cocktails, what happens to the trillions of bricks that make up his body?

The spirits go through the digestive system from the mouth to the stomach and into the intestines, where they are changed into ethyl alcohol. This chemical is then absorbed into the bloodstream. From here it goes into the liver, where it is detoxified into harmless carbon dioxide and water. The capacity of the liver to detoxify alcohol is about half a glass of spirits or one glass of wine per hour. If more than this amount is forced into the liver, it is overburdened. The toxic alcohol overflows and is then transported to the heart, whence it is pumped throughout John Jones's body. All the trillions of bricks are more or less poisoned, but the brain bricks seem to have an affinity for alcohol. As a result, it concentrates more in that area. Then Mr Jones is sick! He cannot articulate clearly, he loses his equilibrium because his muscle bricks are poisoned, and he is emotionally upset because his nerve bricks are also toxic.

If John Jones continues this behaviour over a period of years, a large number of his liver bricks will be destroyed, and he will have a disease known as cirrhosis of the liver. His kidney bricks are also affected, resulting in nephritis. If John Jones's heart bricks are also injured, chronic myocarditis and cardiac decompensation will develop. Other parts of the body are affected in the same manner, and if enough of these trillions of bricks are weakened and destroyed, death occurs.

The sequence of events caused by alcohol is duplicated when the body takes in other poisonous substances, such as microbial agents (bacteria and viruses), and chemical additives in foods.

## Diseases caused by dietary indiscretion

Although the purpose of food is to maintain and sustain life by giving the body necessary nutrition, dietary indiscretion has been practised by affluent nations from time immemorial.

Food is utilised not only as a symbol of wealth but also for social intercourse. Even today in our advanced, intelligent, scientific world, food is used in the same imprudent and uninhibited manner of the Roman Empire before its downfall. Sybaritic living is one of the great human failings.

The inhuman routine of 'a good breakfast', coffee break an 'adequate' lunch, snacks, cocktails, gourmet dinners and constant nibbling while watching television has created a desperate medical problem in this world of abundance. A quarter of our food goes into nourishment, and three quarters into making us ill.

Scientific studies over the past three decades have definitely shown that what we eat can cause such degenerative diseases as heart disease, strokes, diabetes and hypertension. A degenerative disease, according to *Dorland's Medical Dictionary*, '. . . occurs when there is a chemical change of the tissue from a normal to a less functionally active form.' These disorders account for seventy per cent of the annual death rate in the United States, a number that is growing at an ever-increasing speed.

American Government reports indicate that in 1974 over a million people died of heart and vascular diseases, and approximately twenty million people have diabetes, twenty-six million are suffering from hypertension, ten million suffer from asthma, and a million have gout.

These figures evoked the concern of the US government, and recently a national conference was called by the United States Committee on Nutrition and Human Needs, where every aspect of nutrition in relation to diseases was debated, discussed and pondered. The conclusion of this conference was startling:

'We are a nation of nutritional illiterates. A large part of the population takes its opinion about nutrition from advertising, much of that being misinformation, appealing to the eye and taste rather than to a sense of nutritional value. Many of our serious diseases can be attributed to this dietary ignorance.'

## The well-balanced Western diet

Why are we labelled 'nutritional illiterates'? What sort of diet are we eating now? What sort of diet do the medical and nutritional authorities recommend? Let's see what the widely taught 'well-balanced diet' means. Since this book is mainly concerned with rheumatic diseases, here is what is recommended in the American Arthritis Foundation's booklet, *Diet and Arthritis*:

'All the foods any arthritic needs can be found in local food markets – but there is overwhelming evidence that nutritionally balanced meals eaten regularly benefit anyone's overall health and muscle tone, and in the case of arthritis, build ability to resist the wear and tear of the disease. Although some minor adjustments in specific items may be required, in general the good diet for anyone, whether you have arthritis or not, is based on selection from four food groups. Briefly, they are the milk group; the meat group; the vegetable and fruit group; and the bread and cereal group. (1) The milk group: use two or more cups of milk, or its equivalent daily; (2) the meat group: use two or more servings daily; (3) the vegetable and fruit group: use at least four servings of vegetables and fruits daily; (4) the bread and cereal group: use four or more servings daily.'

If the above advice is beneficial, then every citizen should have relatively good health. Why, then, the continuous increase in so many chronic and degenerative diseases that are not caused by germs or viruses? And, if the so-called well-balanced diet is the main factor leading to such degenerative diseases as heart trouble, hypertension, strokes, diabetes and even cancer, doesn't it seem logical to suppose that improper diet may lead to another degenerative disease, namely arthritis?

Not to those in the Arthritis Foundation. Other researchers hint at nutrition's relationship to arthritis, but, perhaps out of timidity they are reluctant to encroach upon the preserves of the foundation, which specifically denies that there is any relationship between diet and arthritis.

Let's look more closely at some specific items in this 'well-balanced diet' and see what scientists have discovered.

## Milk and dairy products

The American Federal Trade Commission is bringing the California Milk Producers' Advisory Board to task for the milk advertising all over the nation. The commission's complaint challenges those familiar claims that 'Everybody needs milk', and 'Milk has something for everybody', and states that for some people milk might be downright harmful.

In the 11 March 1975 issue of the *National Enquirer*, Dr Kurt A. Oster, Chief of Cardiology at Park City Hospital, Bridgeport, Connecticut, said: 'Homogenised milk is one of the major causes of heart diseases in the United States. The fat in the milk contains a substance called xanthine oxidase, or XO, an enzyme. This enzyme will attack the heart and its arteries if it enters the bloodstream; and it is able to get into the bloodstream from homogenised milk.

'When old-fashioned, non-homogenised milk is drunk, the body excretes the XO like any other waste. But when milk is homogenised, the break-up of the fat allows the tiny particles of XO to go through the walls of the intestine into the bloodstream and reach the heart and artery tissues.

'The XO acts chemically to scar the artery walls and heart tissue. The body tries to repair the damage by raising the cholesterol level of the blood, and depositing protective fatty material on the scars. If the process continues, the fatty material begins to clog the arteries, causing heart disease.

'Homogenised milk is the main reason why the United States' cardiac death rate is the highest in the world, next to Finland's.'

Dr Kurt Esselbacher, Chairman of the Department of Medicine of the Harvard Medical School, said: 'I am in full support of Dr Oster's overall concept. Homogenised milk, because of its XO content, is one of the major causes of heart disease in the United States.'

Dr Oster further claimed: 'The foundations of heart

trouble start early in most Americans, because children drink so much milk. The damage caused by XO is a long-term process. The XO builds up in the body. The first ten to fifteen years, when most children drink a lot of milk – that's when the real damage is done.'

The results of autopsies performed during the Korean and Vietnam wars on deceased soldiers substantiated the above statement. Several hundred autopsies were performed, and in half the cases a heart disease called atherosclerosis was found in the coronary arteries. These young men ranged in age from nineteen to thirty.

At a recent meeting of the American Public Health Association, Dr George Christakis, formerly nutritional chief of New York's Mount Sinai School of Medicine, stated: 'Forcing an infant to empty his bottle of cow's milk, and allowing a youngster to join in the McDonald generation, fuelled by hamburgers, malted milk and French fries [chips], can set the stage for chronic diseases in later life. One-third of all American men between the ages of twenty and fifty have high cholesterol levels and are high-risk heart attack possibilities.

'Cow's milk is ideal for calves. It has three times the protein of human milk, but it is not as digestible for a human. It is high in saturated fat, not absorbed as well by the human infant. It is not the perfect food for humans. It was designed for the calf which doubles its weight in fifty days, while the human does this in one hundred and fifty days. . . . Making the nation nutritionally aware means changing the American way of eating at every level.'

Dr Douglas H. Sandberg, Associate Professor of Pediatrics at the University of Miami School of Medicine, said: 'Milk isn't well tolerated by large segments of the world population. This is particularly true of the non-white majority. Some studies show that as many as seventy per cent of blacks do not digest it properly. In spite of this information, milk continues to be a major food in school free-lunch programmes. Many Negro children who participate in these programmes get enough lactose a day to cause them to have such symptoms as abdominal pain and diarrhoea.' Dr

Sandberg recommended that if such symptoms were found to be prevalent in black children drinking milk, it should be eliminated from school lunches and another protein source substituted.

## Saturated fats

Dr Paul Leren, Professor of Medicine at Oslo University, has produced convincing evidence that a change in diet can prevent heart disease. He had a group of 412 middle-aged men (from the ages of forty-four to sixty-four), who had a history of one previous heart attack. The question to be answered was: can a second heart attack be prevented if the patient eliminates animal fats from his diet?

Dr Leren divided these patients into two groups: 206 of his subjects were put on a diet that contained no cream, whole milk, butter, fatty meats, such as beef, lamb, or pork, or egg yolks – almost the Dong Diet. These people were not given any sort of medication. The other 206 subjects continued to eat what they'd always eaten.

Dr Leren kept track of these people for five years, and at the end of the period the score stood like this: among the 206 dieters there were 43 heart attacks in all. Among the non-dieters, there were 64 heart attacks in the group. Ten of the dieters died; 23 of the non-dieters died. In summary, a diet relatively free of animal fats seems to prevent coronary heart attacks.

Dr Jeremiah Stamler, an eminent heart researcher from Chicago, while participating in the American Congress of Cardiology, said: 'The opulent, high-fat, heavy-smoking life of the American may be a far more widespread cause of death from heart disease than race, genetics or even high blood pressure.' Dr Stamler feels the problem is the way that we define the 'good life – our well-marbled steaks, our whipped cream and buttery cakes and our cigarettes'.

The American Heart Association, after analysing data and the results of experiments with the so-called well-balanced diet over the past two decades, has seen its detrimental effects. The association published a cookbook to counteract the misconception underlying the Western way of eating. On the jacket of this book is the astute remark: 'The reason for being, and your reason for using it – are as basic as the most basic recipe in its pages. More than a million Americans die annually from heart and circulatory problems. The foods that we eat, especially fatty foods, are one of the risk factors in heart disease. Our diet is one factor we can do something about.'

The American Heart Association's low-fat, low-cholesterol diet is also approved by the Food and Nutrition Board of the United States National Academy of Sciences–National Research Council and the Council on Foods and Nutrition of the American Medical Association, which also recommended it in a joint statement in July 1972.

Diet is now suspected as being the cause of certain types of cancer. There is little doubt, for example, that our diet is somehow related to the risk of getting colon-rectal cancer. Recently one study has put the spotlight on beef. Other research is indicating fat. One theory pinpoints refined flour and the lack of roughage.

At the moment, the linking of colon-rectal cancer with the diet is largely statistical. For some time, researchers have been mystified by the fact that there are definite geographical differences in death rates from this form of cancer. Since cancer occurs in the bowel, the scientists' first attempts to explain these geographical differences have focused on the dietary differences between the countries.

The results strongly indicate that the researchers are on the right track. For instance, among the Japanese who migrated to Hawaii in 1920 and 1930 and are now in the age groups where colon-rectal cancer is the most common, it was found that the colon-cancer rate is much higher than the rate in Japan, though not as high as the overall United States rate.

A study was made to see if the rate among the Hawaiian Japanese had anything to do with their switching away from the traditional Japanese diet of vegetables and fish to the meat-heavy, fat-heavy American diet. Drs William Haenszel, John W. Berg and others at the American National Cancer

Institute, found that the Japanese immigrants who developed the malignancy had a history of eating considerably more beef than did those of their fellow immigrants who did not develop the disease.

Dr Berg said: 'There is now substantial evidence that beef consumption is a key factor in determining bowel cancer incidence.'

Another frequent cause of death in the West is 'strokes'. A stroke is caused by a blockage of the arteries leading to the brain. Dr John S. la Due of the Sloan-Kettering Institute for Cancer Research in New York City, explaining how this happens, warned against diets rich in saturated fats because such foods interfere with the machinery in the blood vessels that is designed to dissolve blood clots.

### Sugar

Some of the most serious diseases are caused by too much sugar consumption. In the US the annual consumption of sugar per capita is over one hundred pounds. Americans spent approximately two and a half billion dollars on sweets in 1974, and now that sugar prices are so inflated, this sum could possibly rise to seven billion dollars in 1975. Further statistics show that each year the average American consumes about twenty pounds of ice cream and twenty-five gallons of soft drinks – and that soft-drink consumption is increasing by ten per cent each year. This habit has caused three of the most common diseases in the United States – dental caries, or decay, which costs billions of dollars for dental health care annually; diabetes, which afflicts millions of Americans; and obesity, the embarrassing and detrimental disease that is now the scourge of Western society. Figures for Great Britain are not available, but experts agree that, proportionately, they are fast catching up.

### Alcohol

Another disease on the upsurge as a result of luxurious living is liver disease, caused by the excessive use of alcohol.

Figures show that forty gallons of beer, wine and spirits were imbibed per capita in the United States in 1974. This total is rising by about ten per cent annually.

Inadequate sexual performance in men has even been linked to excessive use of alcohol, according to an article in the Chicago *Tribune*.

'Infertility, impotence and feminine characteristics were found in nearly all thirty-seven men with alcoholic liver disease in a new study conducted at Boston City Hospital.

'The latest findings blame alcohol-induced damage to the two sex-controlling glands at the base of the brain.

'The glands – the pituitary and the hypothalamus – produce hormones called IH and PH. These enable the testicles to manufacture sperm and testosterone (the male sex hormone).

'Sixty-eight per cent of the men in the study, age twenty-nine to sixty-five, had markedly reduced levels of testosterone. All had decreased sperm levels, and only one man had normal seminal fluid.'

## Pervasiveness of chemical additives

Because we in the West are always in a hurry for everything, the processed-food industry has grown enormously in the last fifteen years. Supermarkets in the United States sell over 30,000 different kinds of foodstuffs, grossing about 130 billion dollars a year. Manufactured and processed packaged-food items in the form of snacks and convenience foods use over a billion pounds of chemical additives annually – about five pounds per person. Their purpose is to enhance the taste, and the colour, to preserve, to thicken, to acidify and to sweeten. Many of these chemicals are dangerous, untested and absolutely unnecessary, and are suspected causes of many major and minor medical problems, such as severe allergic reactions, gastro-intestinal complaints, asthma, migraines and brain damage, as well as possibly causing carcinoma (cancer). The statistics I have used here are from American sources – but the rest of the Western World cannot be far behind.

## Nitrite

Of nitrite, one of the most dangerous additives, an article in the American publication *Medical World News*, 7 September 1973, said: 'This additive, believed by critics to be the most toxic chemical in the nation's food supply, occurs in most hot dogs, bacon, ham, luncheon meats, smoked fish and related products. Each year more than seven billion pounds of these foods receive nitrite treatment. In cured meats, nitrite acts as a preservative, a flavouring, and a colour fixative that gives them their customary bright pink colour. The present-day use of sodium nitrite stems from the time-honoured use of saltpetre (potassium nitrate) in cured meats. Early in the current century, scientists found that sodium nitrite was a more effective agent . . . but there have been numerous human deaths from accidental nitrite poisoning, giving this substance the dubious distinction of being the only food additive known to have caused fatalities.

'Nitrites, in the presence of stomach acid and secondary or tertiary amines, can form powerful carcinogens [cancer-causing substances] known as nitrosamines.'

## Monosodium glutamate (MSG)

Millions of pounds of this chemical food additive are used annually to intensify the taste of food. Most of the restaurants throughout the United States add it to steaks, chops, fish, soups and salads. So much MSG is used in Chinese restaurants that the resultant symptoms that result such as headaches, diarrhoea, dermatitis and burning sensations in the neck, forearm and chest, are now known in America as the 'Chinese restaurant syndrome'.

The above-mentioned *Medical World News* article said this about MSG: 'Subcutaneous injections of MSG damaged the central nervous system of infant mice and rats . . . along with brain damage, researchers found that some experimental animals suffered from dwarfing and obesity, learning deficits, behavioural disturbances and retinal defects.'

## Food colouring

The article also commented on food colourings: 'Dyes made of coal-tar derivatives are now going into the nation's foods at the rate of about four million pounds annually. A dozen of the dyes have been banned since 1919, when time-honoured "butter yellow" was found to be highly toxic and carcinogenic . . . at present, red No. 2 (amaranth) is the most widely used and highly suspect of the coal-tar dyes going into food. In 1971, the FDA certified for use more than 1.2 million pounds of the dye, which produces the vivid cherry hue of soft drinks and is also added to ice cream, candies, baked goods and sausages. A popular sugar-coated cornflake is sprayed bright pink with red No. 2 and promoted to children as an energy-packed breakfast.'

## What can we do about additives?

As you can see from the above documentation, the pervasiveness of chemical additives in practically all of our modern foodstuffs certainly does not contribute to good nutrition, and research and actual experience have shown them to be health liabilities of both immediate and future concern.

The medical community has started issuing warnings to the public, giving unequivocal evidence that many diseases are caused by dietary indiscretion. Newspapers, magazines and medical journals are used as media to advise the public to change their eating habits. However, diet means restriction and deprivation of certain foods, and psychologically that is unacceptable to the public. We are already living in a world full of regulations and laws, and almost the only remaining 'pleasure' in one's life that has no restrictions is one's eating habits. So most people ignore the warnings and continue eating as they always have.

However, the warnings of both the American Food and Drug Administration and medical scientists everywhere have made many in the food industry conscious of this problem. Products are being put on the market that are free of chemical contaminates.

All of us should support these products and be critical label-readers – not only for our own immediate safety, but to spur others in the industry to follow suit, so that future generations will be protected from the possible harmful effects of the chemical contaminates.

## Medical schools lack nutrition courses

Now that so much information is available on the many diseases caused by nutritional transgressions, why has the medical profession neglected to provide proper diets for their patients, not only as a means of treating present illnesses, but to prevent future illnesses? The answer is provided by Dr Stanley N. Gershoff, Associate Professor of Nutrition at Harvard University, who said at a recent seminar: 'We found a stream of literature on nutrition that was lousy science. We found hardly a medical school where nutrition is being seriously taught, and hardly any real-life nutrition education going on anywhere – not to the public, not to the professionals, not even to the doctors or medical students.' Another member of the seminar group substantiated this statement. Dr Dorris H. Calloway, Professor of Nutrition at the University of California at Berkeley, said: 'Even here at the University of California's prestigious San Francisco Medical Center, there is no regular nutrition course for the medical student, and the only full-time nutrition educator is on the Nursing School staff.'

In the January 1970 issue of the *Medical Tribune*, Dr Jean Mayer, an associate of Dr Gershoff, stated: 'Our studies at Harvard among residents suggest that the average physician knows a little more about nutrition than the average secretary – unless the secretary has a weight problem. Then she probably knows more than the average physician.'

Another critic of the present-day Western diet and its morbid consequences is Dr Alfred D. Klinger, Professor of Preventive Medicine at Rush Medical College, Chicago, who wrote in the August 1974 issue of the *Medical Times*: 'Malnutrition in this country is a malady of the first rank and is responsible in large degree for the high incidence of congenital mental retardation, epilepsy and cerebral palsy; the high prematurity rates and the seventy-five per cent of all infant mortality which results from it in the first month of life; the considerably higher rates of maternal morbidity; the persistent tuberculosis, bone and joint disease, heart condition and hypertensive problems which flower from it.

'Yet there is little or no teaching of and even less interest in nutrition, and little teaching of it in most medical and health professional schools. This is the most tragic part of the spectacle. There are those in the high circles of medicine who are agape at such a thing as malnutrition in the United States. They either deny it, or maintain that only food faddists are susceptible, or will tell you that not enough is known for anything to be done about it.

'As a consequence hardly any doctors know about nutrition. Few take interest in their dietary history or understand how to prescribe a proper diet or to correct one that is improper. Yet nutrition is the cornerstone of life. Its proper application sustains the body and the mind. Its neglect tends to cripple them.'

### Lack of nutrition training in medical schools affects doctors' lives

The truth of Dr Klinger's statement: 'Nutrition is the cornerstone of life. Its proper application sustains the body and mind. Its neglect tends to cripple them,' is manifested daily.

On one day headlines in the newspapers tell of millions dying in India of famine because of crop failures. On another day a headline states that in America over one million people are dying annually of heart and vascular diseases due to the affluent American dietary habits. These two extremes – too little and too much food – can each cause death.

Yet very few medical schools in the United States and Europe have recently added nutrition courses to their curricula for embryo doctors, the people who are being trained to guard our health and lives. They are launched into the practice of medicine without any knowledge of the science of nutrition. Let's see how this lack of training affects the doctors' own lives.

Dr Emanuel Cheraskin, with a research team at the University of Alabama School of Medicine, made a study of the health of 832 doctors and their spouses over the last eight years in five American cities. He came to the conclusion that a doctor's own bad habits may influence the medical advice that he or she gives to you. The doctor who smokes is not likely to be as hard on you about the health hazards of smoking. If the doctor is fat, his or her attitude towards you if you have a weight problem will be different from that of a thin doctor. If the doctor hates to exercise, you will be less likely to learn that physical exercise can improve your health. Similarly, if the doctor does not have much knowledge of nutrition, he cannot advise you on dietary problems. As a matter of fact, most doctors do not have any specific diets that they follow. They usually eat whatever is put in front of them. As a result, they and their spouses develop the same biochemical problems. For example, in the study, male doctors with high cholesterol levels tended to have wives with similar high levels. Dr Cheraskin said: 'The similarities existed all across the board with marital similarities showing up in studies on blood sugar, enzymes, hormonal balance and urine. I found that couples develop similar blood pressure levels after fifteen years of marriage.' It was also discovered that the majority of the people in the study were overweight, and the most prevalent excuse they gave for this condition was that it was a question of genetics. 'This introduced an element of hopelessness,' Dr Cheraskin states. 'The fact is that in those families everybody was eating like pigs.'

### How the lack of training in nutrition affected my life

In 1931, I graduated from medical school without any training in the science of nutrition. I had given very little thought or consideration to the problem of food and its effect on the human body except that I knew that I had to eat to live and work. During the first two decades of my life I had subsisted on a more or less simple Chinese diet, consisting mainly of beef, pork, chicken, fish, vegetables and rice, and never any desserts. However, when I started to practise medicine at the age of twenty-eight, I gradually changed to a diet like that of most Americans. My usual breakfast was orange or tomato juice, ham or bacon with eggs, coffee with sugar and cream; for lunch, it would be such things as tinned soup, roast beef, hot breads, sandwiches, apple pie, all washed down with a soft drink; for dinner I usually ate out at restaurants in the city. In fact, I was eating like a pig!

After seven years I had gained over forty pounds and had developed arthritis. For three years my only relief from the agony of this disorder was the large doses of aspirin and other analgesics prescribed for me by my doctors. In addition to the racking pains in my various joints and muscles, I developed a general dermatitis as a result of an allergy to the medication.

Several diagnoses were made of my condition, among them rheumatoid arthritis, erosive osteoarthritis and psoriatic arthritis. Laboratory facilities at that time were not as sophisticated as they are today, so the doctors were unable to make a more definitive diagnosis.

My condition became progressively worse, and the last doctor I consulted, like all the others, was in a quandary. His final advice was that I should consult a psychiatrist.

I knew that I was slowly going crazy, but I wanted to think that I was not yet ready for the head-shrinker. In my desperation I remembered what my father had said to all of his nine children whenever any of us became ill: '*Bing chung how yup, woh chung how chut.*' Literally translated, this means: 'Sickness enters through the mouth, and catastrophe comes out of the mouth.'

I had forgotten this sage folk observation in my pursuit of Western higher education and scientific knowledge. Now that all the expertise of the West had failed me, I was looking for answers elsewhere and everywhere. Perhaps I had been putting the sickness of arthritis into my mouth for a long time without realising it! Thus this ancient Chinese axiom was the revelation that eventually rescued me from a wheelchair. It pointed me in another direction, away from the orthodox method of treatment.

As an experiment, I went back to the Chinese 'poor-man's diet' that I had been brought up on. I finally settled on seafood, vegetables and rice as the best diet for me. To my utter amazement, in a few short weeks there was a metamorphosis. I was able to shave again, for my skin had become soft and pliable and did not weep. I was agile again, for I went from 14 stone to 11 stone the weight that I maintain today. I was able to play golf again, for the stiffness and pain in my joints disappeared. I was able to smile again, for the psychological torture of years was alleviated. I had almost a complete remission from my crippling disease, which has miraculously lasted until the present day.

My dramatic recovery convinced me that rheumatic diseases are caused by chemical poisoning from the chemical additives put into our food to enhance taste, smell, colouring and for preserving; and by allergy to certain foods.

Upon returning to my medical practice, I combined my newly acquired knowledge of nutrition with a moderate amount of chemical therapy as a working hypothesis to treat all my patients with rheumatic diseases, and I have continued this to this day. I give them a lecture on the subject of nutrition in relation to health and illness. I warn them against the hazards of eating processed and prepared foods containing artificial flavourings, colours, chemical preservatives and other additives. The benefits of these few minutes of conversation with my patients are immeasurable in terms of getting their cooperation and confidence. In the past thirty years or more, I have successfully treated thousands of cases of rheumatic diseases, and had the reward of seeing a high percentage of my patients experience remission from pain and misery.

# 2

# Arthritis:
## types, causes, treatments

Now that you understand what your body is made of, what happens to the food that you eat and what diet and nutrition mean, let us discuss arthritis itself. In this chapter I will briefly try to answer questions which most people have about arthritis. What are the most common forms of arthritis? What causes arthritis? How do you treat arthritis? What is it like to have arthritis? If you are puzzled about arthritis, you are not alone. Over the years many theories and approaches have been taken in an attempt to understand this disease. My colleagues are as confused about it as you may be. Here are titles of the nine recent articles out of over a thousand researched for this book on the subject which I believe will demonstrate the fact that arthritis is still an enigma.

'Rheumatoid Arthritis – Overlooked, Underestimated, Confusing'
'Joint Pain, Is it Really Rheumatoid Arthritis?'
'Problems in Rheumatology: Non-Articular Arthritis'
'Twenty-six Essentials to Differentiate Arthritis'
'Arthritis – Curbing the Crippler'
'Pain Pattern in Rheumatic Disorders'
'Low Back Loser Syndrome; Crippled by Pain, Hooked on Medication, Burdened by Bills'
'New Surgery That May Curb Arthritis'
'Physical Diagnosis in Rheumatoid Arthritis: It is More Certain Than X-rays and Laboratory Tests Combined'.

The American Rheumatism Association and the Arthritis

and Rheumatism Council in Great Britain both list over one hundred different arthritic conditions, but I will name and describe the symptoms of only the most common forms of rheumatic diseases. It is important that you remember that self-diagnosis is dangerous. If you recognise some symptoms, do not assume that you have one of the rheumatic diseases. Many disorders have similar symptoms – pain, inflammation and joint involvement – which can be caused by infectious diseases as disparate as hepatitis, tuberculosis, gonorrhoea and measles.

### Rheumatoid arthritis

Rheumatoid arthritis afflicts more than a million people in Great Britain, and five million in the United States, from infants to the elderly. It is the most destructive and crippling form of arthritis. For reasons that are still unknown, it affects three times as many women as men. Rheumatoid arthritis is usually considered a systemic disease – it involves the blood vessels, the muscles, the heart, the lungs, the kidneys and practically every other organ of the body although the joints are the prime target.

The clinical picture is characterised by joint involvement that is inflammatory, chronic, polyarthritic and symmetrical. For instance, if the knuckles of one hand are involved, the knuckles of the other hand become involved next. Usually it does not involve the distal interphalangeal joints which means that the second and third joints of the fingers are affected, but not the ends of the fingers.

In advanced cases of rheumatoid arthritis, the joints may become totally immobilised due to severe inflammation and swelling of the synovial membranes, surrounding tissues and muscles. The mysterious thing about rheumatoid arthritis is that often there is a remission period – that is, all the symptoms sometimes completely disappear for a period of time, only to flare up again as devastatingly as before. Most rheumatoid arthritic patients can avoid serious disability if the disease is treated in its early stages.

In children, this disorder is referred to as juvenile rheumatoid arthritis, or Still's disease after Dr George Still the English physician who was the first to describe it. In America about six in every ten thousand schoolchildren get some form of Still's disease, but eighty per cent recover completely without ill effects. The most alarming complication of Still's disease is that it is one of the very few arthritic conditions to cause blindness. However, with proper treatment this can be prevented.

## Psoriatic arthritis and Reiter's Syndrome

These two diseases are also classified as polyarthritis of unknown aetiology (origin) and have many of the characteristic features and symptoms of rheumatoid arthritis.

## Osteoarthritis

Osteoarthritis, which claims approximately ten million victims in the United States and four to five million in Great Britain, is a degenerative disease – the wear-and-tear disease of the joints. Typically, it attacks those joints that carry the most body weight and so are subjected to the greatest stress, and consequently the spine, the knees and the hips are the ones affected. The wrists, the elbows, the shoulders and the ends of the fingers can also be affected.

Although it has frequently been thought to be an old man's disease, patients have developed osteoarthritis as early as the age of twenty or thirty, as demonstrated by histologic evidence and X-rays. However, the aching, stiffness and creaking of the joints do not appear until middle age. Osteoarthritis is not a systemic disease, but it affects the joints locally and it goes on for years.

In severe cases the disease may destroy the normal structure of the joints. However, this is not very common, and the ends of the bones do not often grow together as they may in advanced cases of rheumatoid arthritis. The worst type of osteoarthritis involves the hips. Until recently this led to permanent crippling but with today's refined and improved prosthetic design and surgical techniques, total hip replacement has given comfort and mobility to many otherwise hopeless cases.

### Ankylosing spondylitis

Ankylosing spondylitis is one of the more common rheumatic diseases and there are approximately a hundred thousand cases in Great Britain, and a million in the United States. It occurs in men ten times as often as in women, and it usually begins in the early twenties and middle age. This is a chronic inflammatory disease. The inflammation most often starts at the sacroiliac joints and gradually spreads up the spine towards the neck. Occasionally, other joints – the shoulders, the hips and the knees – are affected. It differs from rheumatoid arthritis in that the inflammation is normally confined to the spine, and seldom to the joints of the limbs. In severe cases of ankylosing spondylitis the eyes, heart and intestines are occasionally involved. In diagnosing this disease, X-rays of the spine are essential for they reveal the disorder in its very early states as well as in its later progression.

### Gout

Most of us are familiar with gout. We know more about this disease than all the other types of arthritis – yet there are over a million people in the United States suffering from it today. It is called the 'snob' form of arthritis, because it is more common among the wealthy and successful segments of the population.

A caricature of the gourmand King Henry VIII, seen in comic strips, is a picture description of gout that is worth ten thousand words. King Henry is shown as a fat, well-groomed monarch sitting on a great chair with his leg, bandaged and with a big, red, inflamed toe exposed, resting on a footstool. In one hand he holds a large rib of beef and in the other hand a mug of ale.

At a recent seminar in New Zealand I learned that when the native Maoris deserted their traditional fish-and-vegetable diet for the 'white man's' one of beef, lamb, sweets and dairy products, they developed obesity, cardiovascular diseases and numerous cases of gout.

This confirms the long-known fact that gout is a metabolic disease and that dietary transgression is one of its main causes. People with gout and gouty arthritis usually have high uric acid content in their blood. The foods that contain the most uric acid are brains, sweetbreads, kidneys, liver, meat extracts, sardines, anchovies and caviar. Since the consumption of too many alcoholic beverages injures the kidneys and prevents the body from getting rid of the uric acid, people who eat and drink excessively are prone to gout.

The symptoms of gout, inflammation and swelling of the involved joints, make it the most painful of all arthritic diseases. The big toe is usually the target area, but other parts of the body may also become involved. In severe cases of gout, the kidneys can be damaged by uric acid. Kidney stones sometimes form, causing agonising pains and threatening life itself, for the kidney is then unable to eliminate waste products.

Modern research has given us a great deal of knowledge concerning the treatment of gout. The orthodox method today is the use of the following medication: (1) Indocid, Butazolidin and Tandearil (oxyphenbutazone), successful drugs for relieving the acute pains of gout; (2) probenecid, a drug used to increase the elimination of uric acid; (3) allopurinol, a new and effective drug used to reduce the formation of uric acid in the body, which should be taken indefinitely.

The success of these drugs in the treatment of gout has resulted in a tendency among doctors to under-emphasise dietary measures. In my treatment of gout, dietary restrictions are of the utmost importance. Many of my patients are allergic to the medications used to control gout. If those patients whom I have put on a diet stray from it, they come back to my office and say, 'It's too painful to cheat. I've learned my lesson!'

I consider it unnecessary for patients to have to rely on drugs alone for the rest of their lives when the same results can be accomplished by mere discipline.

## Connective-tissue disorders

Connective tissue essentially binds together and is the support of the various structures of the body. There are three types made up of protein fibrils – collagen, reticulin and elastin. Connective-tissue disorders are thought to be due to auto-immunity – a form of allergy. Auto-immunity, as I discuss further in Chapter 4, means that something goes wrong with the antibodies we have in our bodies to protect us from infections, and instead of fighting invading bacteria and viruses, they somehow attack the body's own tissue.

Inflammation, swelling and pain caused by auto-immunity may occur in all parts of the body, including the lungs, the skin, the heart and the kidneys, as well as the joints.

The connective-tissue diseases are:

1. *Systemic lupus erythematosus*. This condition has all the above symptoms and is often mistaken for rheumatoid arthritis although new laboratory techniques have been able to definitively separate these two diseases. Systemic lupus erythematosus attacks more women than men.
2. *Polyarteritis nodosa*. This is an inflammation of the small and medium-size blood vessels throughout the body.
3. *Scleroderma*. In this disease the skin of the patient throughout the body thickens considerably and becomes hard and rigid with pigmented patches. Scleroderma can also involve the heart, the kidneys and the lungs.
4. *Dermatomyositis*. This is also a systemic disease involving the skin, muscles and connective tissue. The skin usually shows swelling and thickening, and the muscles become swollen, tender and weak. Approximmately seventy per cent of the victims of this disease are female, and it usually occurs after forty years of age.

## Non-articular arthritis

Of the fifty million people in America with rheumatic diseases, twenty million are victims of the articular type of diseases previously mentioned – rheumatoid arthritis, osteo-arthritis, ankylosing spondylitis and also collagen diseases (which mainly affect the joints). The other thirty million fall into the non-articular category, which is often called soft-tissue rheumatism. Joint inflammation is not usually present.

The American Rheumatism Association classifies the following conditions as non-articular rheumatism: fibrositis, inter-vertebral disc and low-back syndromes, myositis and myalgia, tendinitis and peritendinitis (bursitis), tenosynovitis fasciitis, carpal tunnel syndrome and others.

From this classified nomenclature you can see that the principal areas of affliction are the muscles, the tendons, the bursae, the joint capsules and other types of fibrous tissues, fat, and nerves. In other words, all the tissues from the head down to the feet are involved. These are the commonest and mildest forms of rheumatic diseases. Also included are such common conditions as bursitis, stiff neck, backaches and muscle spasms. Very few people go through life without having been attacked by one form or another of this group of rheumatic diseases, and most people do not usually consult doctors. They rely on home remedies, which normally take care of the majority of these disorders.

## Modern theories as to the cause of arthritis

Arthritis is not a single disease but a group of more than one hundred disease entities and syndromes. These ailments date back to antiquity – Pleistocene man was found to have had osteoarthritis in his skeletal remains. Well-preserved Egyptian mummies showed that many of those people had rheumatic diseases. Medical books of ancient China mentioned and described arthritis and the use of acupuncture as a mode of treatment. It is natural, then, that physicians throughout the centuries have propounded many theories as to the cause of rheumatic diseases – and have invented multitudes of methods and medicines for their cure.

For some reason, the medical profession in the United States and Europe has been apathetic towards this group of diseases. Only during the past twenty-five years has special attention been given to the study of arthritis, yet it is one of the three main causes of disability. Intensive efforts and huge sums of money are now being expended to discover the cause, prevention, and possible cure of the rheumatic diseases. The greatest efforts are being channelled into the study of rheumatoid arthritis, because it is the second-largest category of the rheumatic group. In the United States alone there are over five million victims. To emphasise the pervasiveness of this disease, think of seven substantial cities completely populated by victims of rheumatic diseases.

Since rheumatoid arthritis is the most crippling form of the inflammatory illnesses, medical scientists feel that if its aetiology or origins can be discovered, other rheumatic diseases will subsequently be conquered.

Of the many modern theories as to the cause of rheumatoid arthritis, the following are the most prominent ones:

1. It is caused by bacteria or viruses.
2. It is due to the abnormality of the body's defence system – the auto-immune theory.
3. It is caused by a combination of the two items above.
4. It is due to psychiatric or emotional factors.
5. It is caused by metabolic and biochemical factors.

## 1. Rheumatoid arthritis is caused by bacteria or viruses

The oldest of the modern theories is the infection theory. At one time it was thought that the same organism that caused tuberculosis was also responsible for rheumatoid arthritis. Thus, gold salt injections, used at that time for the treatment of TB, were also used for the treatment of rheumatoid arthritis. There are diseases that, in a low percentage of cases, can cause arthritis as part of their symptom-complex. Arthritis can be caused by streptococci, gonococci, pneumococci, the syphilis spirochete, tubercle bacilli and other bacteria and this seems to support the infection theory. When the disease is cured, the arthritic symptoms disappear because the toxins (poisons) from the disease are eliminated. Recently a member of my family developed pain and swelling in her joints resembling an acute case of rheumatoid arthritis. She was hospitalised and on thorough examination was found to have hepatitis. In curing her hepatitis, her arthritis symptoms disappeared. This is the reason why people with joint pains should see their own doctor to determine whether the cause is an infectious type of arthritis, or is due to rheumatoid arthritis and other types listed in this chapter, for which no cause has been found to date.

I remember that in 1929, when I was taking my clinical training in medical school, my professor of orthopaedics was one of those zealous scientists who believed that arthritis was caused by a focus of infection. He thought that the infection could be located somewhere else, such as in the gallbladder, the appendix, the tonsils or the teeth. The infectious organism would then somehow enter the bloodstream, localising in the various joints, causing inflammation and resulting in arthritis. It was believed that arthritis could be cured, then, by removing the focus of the infection.

For several years many normal gallbladders, tonsils and appendixes were removed and healthy sets of teeth were extracted in the hope of curing arthritis.

In fact, when I had arthritis, one of my many consultants suggested the removal of all my teeth. Fortunately I did not heed his advice, and I still have my own teeth today.

Many arthritis researchers are looking for a virus, which they think is the cause of arthritis. Many viruses and virus-like particles have been found in the joints of arthritic victims, but none of these viruses has been shown to be the cause of the disease. No micro-organism has been isolated as a causative factor of rheumatoid arthritis.

## 2. Rheumatoid arthritis is due to the abnormality of the body's defence system—the auto-immune theory

This theory postulates that the body's defence system un-accountably reacts against its own tissues in the joints, causing the lining of the joints to become inflamed and damaged. This is called an auto-immune reaction.

This theory as to the cause of arthritis has been accepted as the 'working hypothesis' for research during the past three decades. Most medical scientists believe that the in-citing organism initiating the whole process is a virus that they have not yet found. However, Dr Charles M. Plotz, a famous rheumatologist, stated in the *Medical World News* of April 1974: 'The concept of auto-immunity in rheumatoid arthritis is open to criticism . . . my guess is that the disease really isn't auto-immune, but that some extrinsic factor is involved.' Dr Plotz's concept agrees with my theory. My extrinsic factors are food allergens and chemical additives. (See Chapter 4 for further discussion of this theory.)

## 3. Rheumatoid arthritis is caused by a combination of the above items 1 and 2

Item 1: This theory suggests the following aetiology – that some bacteria invaded the joints, causing damage to the tissue, changing its character, and thus making the defence system 'think' that the tissue is not its own but a foreign body.

Item 2: The defence system then develops antibodies against the joint tissues.

## 4. Psychiatric or emotional factors as the cause of rheumatoid arthritis

One of the most interesting observations in this theory is made by Dr A. Johnson, whose studies suggest that more arthritics may have psychiatric disorders than was previously believed. The following is a quote from *The Geigy Clinical Forum on Arthritis* (this particular case was cited by Dr

Johnson to exemplify those cases of rheumatoid arthritis which bear the closest resemblance to what is known as conversion hysteria): 'One of the more bizarre cases in the annals of rheumatoid arthritis is that of the woman who had been accused by her husband of infidelity and rapidly developed arthritis in the ring finger. This disease soon spread to all of the fingers of both hands.

'Whatever our ultimate knowledge may be about the origins and course of this disease, psychiatric disorders have been diagnosed on a large proportion of the arthritic patients who have been studied comprehensively during the past two decades. Information about this body of data, and associated hypotheses, may be helpful to physicians, particularly in understanding and managing arthritic patients in whom psychological problems are suggested.'

By and large, rheumatologists reject the idea that the psychiatric factor is the main cause of rheumatoid arthritis. Although all doctors who treat chronic diseases recognise that there is always a psychological involvement, the question remains whether it is the cause or the result of the disease.

## 5. Metabolic and biochemical factors as the cause of rheumatoid arthritis

The only theory that has not been investigated to any extent is the one that says metabolic and biochemical factors (for example, food allergens and chemical additives) are the cause of rheumatoid arthritis.

The reason for this in the United States, at least, is that the American Arthritis Foundation, which is our leading authority on the subject of rheumatic diseases, has flatly stated: 'The relationship between diet and arthritis has been thoroughly and scientifically studied. The simple proven fact is: no food has anything to do with causing arthritis and no food is effective in treating or "curing" it.' This view is concurred with in Great Britain.

Yet the next line of the foundation's booklet, *Arthritis – the Basic Facts*, reads: 'The one exception is with gouty

arthritis. Certain foods increase uric acid levels in the body
and should be avoided.'

Isn't this contradictory? If one kind of arthritis is caused
by food, then why not other kinds of arthritis?

If I had not been afflicted with this disease and faced with
the possibility of being crippled for the rest of my life, I
might have accepted their authoritative statements, and
certainly I would not be writing this book.

The Arthritis Foundation has a responsibility to the
American public and to the members of the medical profession who rely upon its pronouncements. It seems to me
that its members may have accepted without proof the
hypothesis that diet has no relationship to arthritis. Their
statement that this relationship has been throughly and
scientifically studied cannot be true. My clinical observations
contradict this. It is to the detriment of the foundation and
of the general public to prevent further research along this
line.

### How doctors diagnose rheumatoid arthritis

Psychological factors play a very important part in our lives.
When medical students are introduced to the study of a new
disease in clinical practice, they frequently relate the disease
to their personal lives. I recall a fellow student who had
kidney trouble when we studied the kidney diseases, lung
trouble when we studied the lung diseases and stomach
trouble when we studied the gastro-intestinal problems.

If you should have some aches and pains after reading the
chapter on rheumatic diseases, don't automatically diagnose
yourself as having arthritis – but perhaps you *should* go to
have that long-neglected physical examination.

But if you have pains, stiffness and inflammation of the
joints over a period of several weeks, don't just take aspirin
or other medication to relieve the pains (as we all see on the
TV commercials) – they may indicate the first symptoms
of rheumatoid arthritis. Do go to see you general practitioner.

When a rheumatoid arthritic patient consults a doctor,

his first complaints will be of pain, stiffness and swelling of several weeks' duration.

What joints are involved, whether the involvement is symmetrical, unusual fatigue, loss of strength, and morning stiffness that lasts for at least a thirty-minute period are all clues in the history of the patient that may indicate rheumatoid arthritis.

## Laboratory examinations

After a thorough physical examination, the patient is sent for a series of laboratory examinations to confirm the clinical findings of the doctor. Normally the erythrocyte sedimentation rate (ESR) is elevated; this is an index of the severity of the arthritis. The latex fixation test is useful in determining the rheumatoid factor in the serum of the patient's blood. The most important of all the laboratory tests is the one that aspirates (draws out) the fluid from the joints for examination. This gives much information to substantiate the rheumatic disease.

Other laboratory tests, such as anti-nuclear antibody test (ANA), total complement test, and immunoelectrophoresis (IEP) test, help the doctor in his differential diagnosis – to distinguish rheumatoid arthritis from other types of arthritis.

In the early stages of rheumatoid arthritis, X-ray examination does not reveal much, but in severe cases of perhaps six months' duration, erosion of the joints will appear in the film.

The history, physical examination and laboratory test results will usually give the doctor a comprehensive picture of the arthritic condition of the patient. He can then proceed with his treatment programme.

## Therapy and management of arthritis

A United States government survey in 1970 showed that the annual direct cost of medical care for arthritic patients in that country was as follows:

|                                          | Cost (in millions |
| Care                                     | of dollars)       |
|------------------------------------------|-------------------|
| Hospitalisation                          | $854              |
| Doctor's consultations                   | 493               |
| 'Quackery' products                      | 408               |
| Prescription drugs                       | 600               |
| Non-prescription drugs                   | 500               |
| Other than physician services            | 50                |
| Federal and private programmes for arthritis | 26            |
|                          Total:          | $2,931            |

In 1966, the same direct cost of medical care had been only a third as much. These statistics also showed that in that year there were seventeen million arthritic victims in the United States, and in less than five years, in 1970, the total had increased to 20,230,000 victims – so, obviously, whatever method of treatment the American medical world is using to prevent and cure rheumatic diseases it is ineffective.

The following treatment programme is the one that is followed by most doctors both in the United States and Europe in the treatment of rheumatoid arthritis:

1. In the beginning stages of the disease, the emphasis is on the relief of pain, prevention of inflammation and deformities and maintenance of function. The family and the patient are warned they must have a long-term outlook towards the treatment. Aspirin is considered the best treatment because it stops the pain and reduces inflammation. Very large doses are given to the patient – as many as twelve to twenty-five tablets a day.

2. If the patient does not respond to the treatment, and the disease continues, becoming moderately severe, affecting multiple joints and causing considerable physical disturbance and disability, then further measures are added to the basic regimen. Other types of medication given are phenylbutazone, indomethacin,

antimalarials and intra-articular steroids. At the same time, intensive physical and occupational therapy and orthopaedic devices, such as splints, bars and canes, are used.

3. If the patient should fail to respond adequately to these measures, then oral steroids and gold treatment are given. There are many side effects to these chemical agents, and some doctors prefer not to use them. Gold is a potent anti-arthritic agent and has been in clinical use for almost fifty years, but its toxicity and side effects are formidable. A blood count, platelet count and urinalysis should be taken frequently while the patient is undergoing gold therapy.

4. About thirty-five per cent of rheumatoid arthritis patients get well with almost no recurrences, about fifty per cent continue to be afflicted, with occasional remissions and recurrences, and fifteen per cent are severe cases and have no remissions at all. Hands, feet and hips then become deformed and crippled, and surgical measures are resorted to for the patient's comfort and function.

5. Those patients who are unresponsive to the conventional therapy are then given experimental medication – immunosuppressive drugs or cytotoxic agents such as cyclophosphamide, chlorambucil, azathioprine, D-penicillamine, histidine, dimethyl-sulfoxide, radioactive gold and aryl acids (mefenamic, fluenamic).

## The drug-oriented West

Although the number of victims of rheumatoid arthritis has gradually increased during the past two decades, the conventional method of treatment has not changed much, except that many new medications have been introduced to treat the symptoms. The present generation of doctors seem to be strongly drug-oriented, their one goal being to find more and better drugs as the panacea for the rheumatic diseases.

Recently a new drug, ibuprofen, was introduced. In a

year-long experiment involving about a thousand patients, ibuprofen showed effectiveness comparable to that of aspirin, but with fewer gastro-intestinal problems. The drug is not a cure – it only suppresses the symptoms like aspirin. A recent check on the cost of ibuprofen in the San Francisco area revealed that the price is seventeen dollars per hundred tablets, while two hundred and fifty tablets of aspirin cost only one dollar. And the chemist mentioned that the pharmaceutical house is already six weeks behind in orders for it.

If there is any need to substantiate the claim that doctors are drug-oriented, the backlog of orders for this new drug shows it clearly. Other companies are hurrying to put out similar drugs.

## Aspirin

In the United States alone about fifteen thousand *tons* of aspirin are produced and consumed annually. Although aspirin is considered a safe drug, the large doses that are prescribed for rheumatoid arthritis patients often create serious consequences.

Dr Harvey J. Weiss, Professor of Medicine at Columbia University, stated in the *Journal of the American Medical Association* of 26 August 1974: 'Ingestion of aspirin, in doses of 1 to 3 grams a day, will induce occult gastro-intestinal bleeding in about seventy per cent of normal subjects. This generally amounts to a daily faecal blood loss of approximately 5 ml (normal loss is less than 1 ml), although much greater losses have been recorded in some individuals. In habitual aspirin users, occult gastro-intestinal bleeding may result in an iron-deficiency anaemia. More serious are the reports that aspirin ingestion can cause acute and massive gastric haemorrhage.

'Aspirin-induced asthma is by far the most serious of the adverse reactions . . . [A small percentage of aspirin takers develop a hypersensitivity, and according to Dr Weiss] . . . death may occur within minutes after ingestion of the drug unless appropriate measures are instituted immediately.

'Aspirin has also been implicated in causing various

types of skin eruptions, transient albuminuria, nephro-
toxicity and thrombocytopenia. In addition, aspirin ranks
second only to barbiturates among drugs used for the purpose of suicide. Aspirin overdose is still a frequent cause of
accidental poisoning in children.'

Since my illness some thirty years ago, when I was given
four to five grams of aspirin a day (equivalent to twelve or
fifteen tablets), I have been reluctant to prescribe any large
doses of aspirin to my patients and I immediately cut down
to the lowest possible dose what they have been taking. In
my opinion, every doctor who prescribes such large doses
to his patients, because some authority said to do it, should
first be made to experiment on himself with fifteen aspirins
a day for a week to see what reactions he gets to this supposedly 'safe' drug. After the week's trial with the aspirin,
I am sure he would be hesitant about prescribing such large
doses to *any* patient over a period of months or years.

## Case histories

In the next few pages I present some case histories of patients
with the various rheumatic diseases who were treated with
my dietary regimen, with moderate doses of medication and
with acupuncture. These cases are typical of those I treat, and
I want to emphasise the fact that every one of my patients
is a chronic case, for all patients who come to my office
are screened. If their arthritis is of recent origin, I advise
them to go to their local doctor or to a specialist for examination and treatment. Only if they have been suffering for
years do I consider them as potential patients, because they
present a challenge to me. Each has had extensive laboratory
tests of every kind and X-rays to substantiate that they are
afflicted with one of the rheumatic disorders. They bring in
histories taken over a period of several years, so that it is not
necessary for me to subject them to further tests unless those
they've had are not of recent date. Each patient also brings
in with him or her vials of coloured pills and vitamins and
aspirin in every form.

I have presented these case histories in an informal manner so the patients can express their own emotions about the problems of their disease. As you read about their personal experiences, you will then understand the problems that typical victims of arthritis face every day of their lives.

Interview taped on 1 March 1974

[*Mrs V. W. is a fifty-seven-year-old housewife who came into my office in March 1973 for the treatment of rheumatoid arthritis. This tape was therefore made one year from the time she started her treatment with me.*]

'Two years ago, while I was playing golf, a golfer on the next fairway sliced a ball and struck me in the chest with it. I was taken to the hospital where they found that I had two fractured ribs. They even thought I had a heart attack. But about a week later, it turned out that I had arthritis in my ribs and not a heart attack, because my left knee started to get swollen and very painful too. Then the pain went up to my hips. My sister, who is a specialist at the University of California Hospital sent me to be taken care of by a rheumatologist. He gave me the whole works, all the examinations, blood work, ECG and all kinds of other tests. He diagnosed my condition as rheumatoid arthritis. He gave me a shot of cortisone in my chest, because that was where I had the severe pains. He also gave me injections in my knees. But the knee got so swollen that they had to drain it twice. My condition became worse, I could not walk up the stairs at all. If the elevator was out in our apartment building I had to stay indoors all day. I could not get in and out of bed by myself. I could not take a bath by myself. It was difficult for me to get in and out of a chair. Riding in an automobile was most painful – I hurt all over. The doctor gave me heavy doses of aspirins, cortisone and Indocid, which helped me some.

'About that time my husband retired, so we decided to move to Coronado, where the weather was better and warmer. My sister recommended another rheumatologist down there to take care of me. I had to go through all the examinations again. This doctor put me on the same medication. My general condition became worse. I had so much pain I could hardly do anything. In addition, I was taking so much cortisone that I acquired an ugly moon face.'

[*The patient was put on the Dong Diet. I explained to her my theory that her rheumatoid arthritis was probably due to food allergy and allergy to the chemical additives in her food. She was admonished to adhere strictly to the diet.*

*Since the patient had been taking large doses of medication for quite a while, it was necessary gradually to decrease the medication as she improved. After two days of dieting, the patient was given four consecutive daily acupuncture treatments in my office.*

*She responded very well to this therapy programme. Her pains decreased and she lost approximately seven pounds. On 29 March 1973, Mrs W. was instructed to return to her home in Coronado to rest, but to keep in touch with me by telephone. A week later she telephoned to tell me that she felt much better and had lost more weight. At this point I instructed her to halve the dosage of her medication. Two weeks later she phoned me to report that her pains had completely disappeared.*

*On 17 May 1973, Mrs W. returned to my office for further treatment. She walked into my office without help. She was pain-free. She weighed ten stone, having lost twenty-seven pounds since I first began treating her.*

*Due to some residual swelling and stiffness in her joints, I continued to give the patient acupuncture treatment on that basis once a month, until 1 March 1974, when the patient was discharged.*]

'Today I weigh nine stone two pounds. During the last five months I have taken about five cortisone tablets only. I used to take five every day, together with about twenty aspirins a day. Now I do not take any aspirins at all. I ride around Coronado on a bicycle and my friends think that I am crazy to go to see a doctor any more. My husband is very proud of me now and said it was just like a new honeymoon.'

Interview taped on 23 August 1974

[*Mrs C. B., aged thirty-nine, a housewife, came into my office for treatments in June 1973, complaining of having been severely ill with rheumatoid arthritis since the age of twenty-one. At that time she started having symptoms of aches and pains in her knees and ankles from time to time. She went to several doctors, who gave her pills to take but made no definite diagnosis. These intermittent pains and aches lasted for about ten years, until one night in 1961, Carol woke up in the middle of the night with a sudden exacerbation of her symptoms.*]

'It was in 1961 when I went to bed one night, perfectly normal with no indication of anything wrong. Then in the middle of the night I was awakened with my hands completely distorted and my arms as stiff as boards and they felt like something was going up and down in them. I was screaming because I had such excruciating pains. Our family doctor was called, and he diagnosed it as muscle spasms. He gave me some pills and told me to stay in bed and rest. I did not get any better, so he finally sent me to a hospital to find out what was exactly wrong with me. After several days they told me that I had rheumatoid arthritis.

'Then they started treatments on me. They gave me medicines and followed up with physiotherapy. I was in and out of the Presbyterian Hospital where they gave me the hot wax treatment on my hands and feet; then at other times they gave me ice packs; you just name it, they tried everything. For starters they gave me thirty aspirins a day, which, needless to say, ruined my stomach. I had repercussions from that and got very sick. So they stopped that treatment and then had me on Darvon. They gave me gold shots also. They must have tried just about every medication that there is associated with this disease. I was sort of a guinea pig for pills. Then they gave me cortisone shots, which also did not work. Finally, they gave me prednisone and Percodan [oxycodone], and also aspirin again, which seemed to be the best combination for me. I had to take these pills all the time in order to stop the stiffness, and the pains and aches.

'In 1962 even though I was still suffering from the disease I married a wonderful man who had stood by me all these years. I could hardly walk down the aisle of the church, for that day was the first time in a year that I wore shoes.

'I was determined to have a baby to make something meaningful of my life and to have someone to share life with. The rheumatologist told us that during pregnancy I might not have any symptoms of the rheumatoid arthritis, but I was not one of the lucky ones. I had to continue with the medication in order to have my baby.

'So we had Lisa, a caesarean baby. It was tough, but we made it. During the six-week check-up, the doctor found that I had cancer of the cervix, so I had to have a hysterectomy. From then on my arthritis became worse, even though I was taking the various medicines. My hands, knees and feet became deformed and I had to have a series of operations.

'My first operation was on my hands, then my knees. In fact, I had both my hands and my knees operated on within six months' time because it was so bad. Then my toes separated from my metatarsal bone and they had to reconstruct one foot, and at the same time they did a double bunionectomy. Then they repaired the tendons of the right foot, hoping that the toes would not separate. After that they asked me to have another operation. This was the straw that broke the camel's back! After going through all those operations they said that I should have my left elbow operated on because of the terrible pains I had in it. They said that it was due to calcium deposits. The only thing that they could do was to go in and scrape the elbow, like they did to my hands. No guarantee that it would be well. I told my husband that I would not have any more surgery.

'Just about that time I heard about Dr Dong and his treatment with arthritis.'

[*Mrs B. was put on the Dong Diet. She was told that she should adhere strictly to the diet plan. She had been taking the following medication, prescribed by her former doctor: Thirty aspirins a day, prednisone (15 mgs), Butazolidin, and Percodan*

*when the pain became too severe. One week later, the patient*
*returned to my office. Prior to her first acupuncture treatment,*
*it was necessary for her to have assistance in undressing. Her*
*husband and my nurse assisted her and the three of us lifted*
*her on to the examination table.*

*She continued to follow her diet rigidly. She was given*
*acupuncture therapy once or twice a month, according to her*
*degree of improvement. Also, her medication was gradually*
*decreased as she began to feel better. The patient lost thirty-*
*two pounds. She was free of pain.*]

'It used to be that I could not even use the vacuum cleaner
without having repercussions for about two days. I have a
great deal of stamina now. In fact, in the autumn of 1973,
my husband and I painted the whole house, inside and
outside.

'I do not take any aspirin now and I only take three
milligrams of prednisone a day, and I am now trying to cut
that down. But I am adhering strictly to the diet. I got off a
few times and got sick. Never again!'

Interview taped on 8 March 1974

[*Mrs A. W. is a thirty-nine-year-old schoolteacher.*]

'I have had rheumatoid arthritis for about ten years, since
1963. While working at the local school, I hit my wrist on a
towel bin and I thought that I had broken it. I had X-rays
taken and they showed that nothing was broken. The pains
went from my wrist down to my knuckles and fingers and
soon my left hand was bothering me and I could not tolerate
the pain at all.

'I decided to come down to San Francisco to go to a good
specialist that we had heard about. This doctor diagnosed it
as rheumatoid arthritis, after extensive examinations. He
told me to take aspirin tablets until I heard bells ring and
then to cut back on the amount of aspirin that I took. That
was about all that he said could be done for it. So I continued on with this treatment, but with constant pains in

various joints and stiffness in my arms and legs, especially in the mornings.

'I became pregnant with my first child. While I was pregnant the problem with the pain went away. My second pregnancy in 1965 was the same way; during the time I was pregnant I had almost no trouble. But after the baby was born, the pain came right back and it got progressively worse. At times my joints would be so inflamed that I would have to crawl around the house. I could not put any weight on them at all; but I had responsibilities with my family and I had to do the work the best way that I knew how, so I continued to take large doses of aspirins in order to be able to do this work.

'In 1969, when the pains became so bad that I could not stand it any longer, I was recommended to see another specialist in San Francisco, a famous rheumatologist. He confirmed that I had rheumatoid arthritis after examining me and repeating many laboratory tests. He decided that I was taking too many aspirins and that there was something better for me. I tried his new medicine for a while, but it did not agree with me. So I went back to the aspirin for pain.

'A new teacher came to school who had arthritis. He had been treated by a doctor in Mexico. Since I was going on vacation with my family in Baja and would be passing through this town in Mexico, I decided to try this method of treatment.

'I consulted with this doctor in Mexico and he gave me medication that I kept on for three years. All the joints went down in size. But after a while, I had some bad reactions. The skin from my knees down to the ankles became very thin and if I knocked my knees on a table or any object that was solid, it would break open like a watermelon. I became very alarmed.

'I went to the University of California Hospital in San Francisco for a week's stay. They told me that it was the massive doses of steroids that I had been taking from the doctor in Mexico. They made me go off these steroids immediately. As I was going off the medication my knees ballooned up and my joints flared up and I even got nodules on my elbows, hard nodules. I was very sick. I could not bend my knees because they were so inflamed. I could not walk up or down the stairs because of the pains. My husband had to get me out of bed in the morning, and also out of anything that was low, like a chair or the car. I could not sit in a chair that did not have arms so I could push or pull myself out of it.

'I consider myself a very capable person, I can do anything that I make up my mind to do, but this rheumatoid arthritis was getting to a point where I was not able to manage for myself. I know that I would have been in a wheelchair if I did not have two children to take care of. I am not the kind of person to give up, but I was very close to the point of giving up after I left the University of California Hospital.'

[*During Mrs W.'s first visit, she was put on the Dong Diet and warned to adhere to it rigidly. She weighed twelve stone and was grossly overweight for her age and height. She was told to restrict her intake of carbohydrates.*

*Her medication had consisted of twenty-four aspirin tablets a day, prescribed by her previous doctor. These did not curb either the pain or the inflammation of her joints. She was almost completely helpless. Subsequently the patient was given one acupuncture treatment a month for six months.*

*The patient responded to the therapy programme amazingly well. She lost three stone and was completely pain-free.*]

'As long as I stay on the diet I feel great. The minute that I deviate either by mistake or otherwise, I find that I have pain and I know it immediately. Now I am back to my teaching job, and I am happy again. I am not taking any medication at all except an aspirin once in a while, when I occasionally get a pain.

'Last week the children of my class and I had a race to the classroom door. That is something that I had not been able to do for ten years.'

## Review and comment

In thinking about these three cases, I am reminded of Shakespeare's sage if unscientific remark; 'Desperate diseases require desperate measures.' The attending physicians on these cases seem to have been carrying this out. The prognosis of all three was practically hopeless. Each woman had been treated by specialists and superspecialists, in clinics and superclinics. Moreover, there were further disadvantages. These patients had been warned by the Arthritis Foundation handbook: 'It is extremely important to understand that the major forms of arthritis are chronic. This means the condition, once started, continues usually for life. It means that one does not "heal up as good as new", as after the common cold, measles or a cut in the skin. It means that whatever damage takes place remains permanently . . . and tends to get worse unless proper precautions are taken to prevent it. It means treatment must continue on and on.'

Was it idiotic of me to try to salvage these hopeless cases when so many specialists had failed? Should I have sent them home with large doses of aspirin to wait for some medical scientist to make the 'breakthrough' that has been promised year after year since 1948, or for the spontaneous remissions that rheumatologists have frequently talked about?

It is now history that these three 'hopeless' cases have recovered from the depths of their mental and physical despair. The victory was attained by the full overall performance and cooperation not only of the patients but also of their families in following the therapeutic programme that I outlined for them.

Now Mrs A. W. is teaching school again and racing the children to the door. Mrs C. B. has painted her house, and Mrs V. W. is riding her bicycle all around Coronado, waving to her friends, who think she is slightly crazy to continue flying up to San Francisco to see her doctor. They feel and act as if they are as good, or better, than ever.

Why didn't these women get well with all the 'supertreatment' that they had received? Why didn't they get that 'spontaneous remission' during all those treatments in the past? I think that the fault lies in the fragmentation of our medical system. Scientific and technological advances in medicine have increased knowledge so extensively that it necessitates the formation of groups of specialists and super-specialists in every field. The drawback of this is that the human body is divided into many parts for the study and treatment of rheumatic diseases, with the result that doctors forget that there is a total human being. A comic once said that when his nose cold went down into his chest, he had to change doctors to cure it. There is a great deal of truth in that statement.

Among the other shortcomings of the treatments that prevented the women's recovery were these three outstanding factors: (1) the patients were not given a sensible dietary programme – they were allowed to put any type of food and drink into bodies that were already enfeebled by their chronic disease; (2) the patients were allowed to acquire another disease – obesity; each one of them gained thirty to forty pounds. This excess weight not only encumbered their already diseased joints but also promoted eventual hypertension, vascular and heart disease, diabetes, and other nutrition-related diseases; (3) large doses of aspirin and other toxic drugs were prescribed over long periods of time. Aspirin, as decribed by Dr Weiss, has many drawbacks. It has caused gastro-intestinal diseases such as ulcers, gastritis, internal bleeding, kidney malfunction, colon ulceration, loss of taste and eye trouble.

Reviewing the entire medical spectrum, the discipline of rheumatology, full of ambiguities and polemics, is surely one discipline that needs a little creative heresy and dissent – for twenty million seriously ill arthritic victims are waiting for a few answers to their agonies instead of twenty aspirin every day.

The American Arthritis Foundation has spent many millions of dollars and many years of research on the rheumatic diseases. Why haven't they reached their goal of 'both prevention and cure'? Possibly because of a long-standing obsession. The elite members, as brilliant young medical students, were bacteriologically oriented, and seemingly they cannot break away from that inculcation. Their whole research programme is geared towards finding some viruses or infectious organisms as the cause of arthritis, or of finding that rheumatic diseases are caused by some over-action of the body's immunity in the defence system, possibly initiated by infection with a virus or a mycobacteria. Probably their research funding for 'young scientists' is earmarked for projects that fit in with their master plan of searching for viruses or bacteria. I suspect that if a young scientist dared to ask for a grant to pursue his own ideas, such as whether or not there is a correlation between nutrition and arthritis, he would be thrown out of the foundation's offices.

I think it was Confucius who said, 'To oppose authoritarianism is not only a strategic necessity but a spiritual imperative.' This is a beautiful philosophy, but to oppose authority is to live in a lonely world – as I, with my dietary hypothesis, have done – and to suffer the indignities of all iconoclasts. But to be able to give a new outlook in life to these three women and others like them is sufficient inspiration for me to continue on with my work. The prolonged suffering of these victims had extended adversely into the lives and life-style of their families and friends. Their recovery has lifted a heavy responsibility and burden from their loved ones, which makes me doubly happy.

These incidents, together with thousands of inspiring letters from all over the country, and now from many of my medical colleagues, have given my spirits a new lift.

# 3

# How the chemicals in our food
# poison our bodies

Let's return for a minute to Fantasyland. Keep in mind the fact that we are made up of sixty trillion bricks and that each one of these bricks is alive and functioning. When John Jones became intoxicated, he overloaded himself with alcohol that his liver could not detoxify. This resulted in the poisoning of trillions of his bricks, which made him drunk, inebriated, intoxicated or whatever term one chooses to describe the mental and physical condition he was in. Perhaps the best word to describe his condition is 'sick'!

Following this logic, my theory and my contention is that the thousands of chemical substances that are routinely added to our foods and absorbed by us cause poisoning and damage to the trillions of joint bricks and other tissue cells surrounding the joints, resulting in a disturbance of function, which we call arthritis. For poison as defined in *Dorland's Medical Dictionary* is 'any substance which, when ingested, inhaled or absorbed, or when applied to, injected into, or developed within the body, in relatively small amounts, by its chemical action *may cause damage to structure or disturbance of function*'. (Italics mine.)

In the case of John Jones, the alcohol had an affinity for his brain bricks, causing his loss of equilibrium. In the case of victims of arthritis, various toxic substances have an affinity for the joint bricks, causing inflammation and disrupting function.

## Arthritis induced by chemicals

Is there any evidence or substantiation that chemicals can cause arthritis?

One serious type of arthritis, systemic lupus erythematosus (SLE), closely related to rheumatoid arthritis, has been induced by several drugs. Remember that drugs are chemicals. One of these chemicals is hydralazine (its trade name is Apresolin), which is used in the treatment of high blood pressure, and there is evidence that this drug has caused this devastating form of arthritis.

Procainamid, another medication used to control abnormal heartbeat rhythm, has also been shown to have caused the same disease. And phenothiazines, a major group of tranquillisers, have been responsible for numerous cases of SLE.

Other medications, such as various antibiotics, have also induced SLE and probably other types of arthritis. The mere removal of these chemicals has spectacularly 'cured' this type of induced disease. These facts are known to the medical profession. It is the direct 'cause–effect–cure' syndrome: a poisonous chemical was ingested – *causing* a pathological condition in the joint bricks – *effecting* a condition called arthritis – and *cured* by not taking any more of the hydralazine, procainamid or whatever chemical the arthritis victim had ingested.

Another example of chemical poisoning resulting in symptoms highly resembling a typical case of arthritis was reported by Dr Gerald T. Perkoff, Professor of Medicine at Washington University, St Louis, Missouri. His report said: 'The changes in the muscles of alcoholics pass through several stages; first there are chemical alterations, then tenderness, then increasingly severe muscle cramps, then a wasting away of the muscle tissue, and finally weakness that is often severe enough to incapacitate the alcoholic totally. It appears more than likely that the alcohol itself is poisonous to the muscle cells.'

Dr Perkoff went on to say: 'In the chemical changes the muscle cells lose large amounts of vital protein called myoglobin, which normally serves to carry oxygen into the muscle tissue. Under the electron microscope the leaking muscle cells separate into weakened fibres, and also show dangerous swellings. When the muscle disease comes on suddenly, it goes just as fast – after a few days or weeks in a hospital with no alcohol and good nutrition. But it will come back if the patient starts drinking again. Patients whose muscle disease has persisted for a long time, however, are much harder to treat; it may take months before their strength returns.'

Here again is a 'cause-effect-cure' syndrome.

Put in my terms, when the poisonous alcohol injured the muscle bricks, it caused the loss of a large amount of myoglobin. As a result, the victim started to have severe muscle cramps due to oxygen deficiency. Under the electronic microscope Dr Perkoff saw that the leaking muscle bricks were broken into pieces and the whole structure began to swell. When the patient is confined in a hospital and pre-vented from putting the poison into his body, the trillions of muscle bricks regenerate themselves and he recovers. But let this person ingest the poison again, and this same symptom complex recurs.

This experiment by Dr Perkoff is important to my theory because certain other very serious forms of arthritis, poly-myalgia rheumatica, polymyositis and dermatomyositis, have symptoms very similar to those he studied.

Let us consider this case history from my own files.

[*Mrs A. P., a 50-year-old office worker came into my office complaining of pains in both of her shoulders and hips. These pains radiated down both arms and both legs. Mrs P. had been treated by her own doctor and also by a specialist. They gave her a series of tests and diagnosed her problem as polymyositis.*]

'This trouble started in July 1973, and I first thought I had the flu because I had pains in all my joints and muscles. I took some aspirin and after two days the pains went away. But soon afterward the pains came back – only worse than before. They were in my shoulders, arms, legs, thighs, the tips of my fingers and the tips of my toes. I felt like I was paralysed.

'In the mornings I had the feeling that I had been poisoned and felt unusually fatigued. The doctors had given me pills to take and I was not getting any better. I was vomiting and feeling worse each day. I was failing instead of being helped.'

[*Mrs A. P. was sent to me by one of my patients. She was put on the Dong Diet. The patient had been taking approximately fifteen aspirins a day and five mgs of Valium twice a day for her nervousness. As the aspirins did not seem to relieve her pains, I prescribed Darvon (sixty-five mgs) three times a day. She was told to continue with the Valium.*]

'After only a week I began to feel better and now two months later, all the pains are gone. I have not felt like this since I was eighteen years old. I have been strictly on the diet – no fooling around or cheating. I have fish with all my meals, even in the morning before I go to work. I bought a *wok* and cooked Chinese-style food. I do not want any more of these pains, so I am following the diet absolutely.'

[*Mrs A. P. does not take any medication at the present time.*]

In the *Primer on the Rheumatic Diseases* compiled by the Arthritis Foundation, polymyositis and dermatomyositis are defined as 'diffused inflammatory disorders of striated muscle . . . these are perplexing disorders of unknown cause, which occur in all age groups, and are usually grouped with the connective tissue diseases . . . the classical rash of dermatomyositis occurs in about forty per cent of patients with inflammatory myopathy.'

Polymyositis, then, is an inflammation of many muscles of the body – and dermatomyositis is the same disease, inflammation of the muscles, accompanied by dermatitis, or skin rash, in about forty per cent of the cases.

I do not know what poisonous substances or how much Mrs A. P. might have ingested, but whatever they were, the allergens were in her food and they created the same onset of symptoms as Dr Perkoff's alcoholic had – aches, pains, stiffness and fatigue. Her doctors had diagnosed her condition as polymyositis, on symptoms and laboratory tests. Such tests show an excess of muscle enzymes in the blood, that can be detected and measured and which indicated muscle destruction. Trillions of her muscle bricks, then, were insulted, damaged and destroyed.

In polymyositis, the toxic substance carried by the blood vessels attack only the muscle bricks, breaking them to pieces and causing the inflammation. But in dermatomyositis, in addition to attacking the muscle bricks, some of the poison goes into the skin bricks, causing severe inflammation of the skin, or dermatitis. Now you may ask: why doesn't the poison attack everyone in the same way? The answer is that human beings are unique – no two individuals are alike, no two fingerprints are alike, no two sets of teeth are alike. Therefore, when people are poisoned, there are qualitative and quantitative differences due to the strength and natural resistance of each brick or group of bricks.

## Two typical cases of arthritis treated by my diet

Mrs C. C., aged seventy-five, gave me the following story on her first visit to my office on 7 March 1974. She was already on the Dong Diet which she had learned about through my book.

'I had been suffering with arthritic pains in my shoulders, back, neck and hips for approximately five years. I was treated at one of the large hospital clinics by several doctors. The pain seemed to be the most severe in both of my hips, and the only relief that I got was going to the hospital to get Novocain shots to quell the pains. The attacks would vary from one to three months and in between times I just toughed it out. When the pains became too unbearable, my son would put me in a wheelchair and take me to the hospital to get these shots.

'About three years ago I was not satisfied with all these shots and not getting any better. So I went to a private rheumatologist. After much examination, he diagnosed my arthritis as progressive osteoarthritis. He said there was no hope for a cure. It came with old age. Taking aspirin was all he said that I should do as the other drugs were too strong for me at my age. I continued with this doctor until I heard about the diet.

'Within a couple of weeks – that seems such a short time now, but I am sure that it was just that – I started to get relief from the pains. And after a couple of months, I was experiencing a return of youthful strength in spite of my age. By January I would have flashes of strength that I would just sit and enjoy, it was so wonderful. It was just like a burst of sunshine through the clouds. Just youthful energy. I have not been in a wheelchair since going on the diet. I just get a twinge of pain here and there once in a while that shows me that I may have veered away from the diet a little. Then I search within myself to see what I might have eaten that was wrong. Eliminating that particular food would then clear up the pains.'

Mr P. E., the second case, also learned of the diet through my book, and wrote to me about his experiences on 13 September 1974.

'It was just a year ago that the pain, swelling and stiffness in my ankles and feet was so bad that I would be awake in tears at night. Actually the problem of aching feet started in May 1973; by September I was on crutches, unable to walk. I went to see a local orthopaedic specialist who felt the problem was rheumatoid arthritis and suggested I see an internist to make certain that there was nothing else causing the pain. The internist concurred with the rheumatoid arthritis diagnosis but sent me to a rheumatologist for further examination. I was placed on a regimen of 20–25 Ecotrin (spare the stomach and good-bye intestines!) and a cortisone derivative daily. After a few weeks of continuing pain, I entered hospital for a month of exhaustive testing and bed rest (and more Ecotrin). [Ecotrin is a brand of aspirin.]

'After being discharged I walked about ten city blocks to have a prescription for orthopaedic shoes filled, and by the

time I arrived there I felt like I had before I went to the
hospital.

'I stayed in contact with the internist by telephone and he
altered the medication dosages (sort of like roulette), but to
no avail. After three more weeks of worsening pain, along
with a bonus of muted hearing, dizziness and hot flashes, I
heard of *The Arthritic's Cookbook*, which I purchased at a
nearby bookshop. As per instructions I threw away the pills,
went on the diet, and thanks to the loving care and attention
of my wife, and the diet (to which she also adheres), I am
now completely relieved of all pain and discomfort. I'm on
my feet twelve to fourteen hours daily with no problems
whatsoever. I'm forty years old, but my body feels as it did
when I was twenty.'

### Commentary on the above two cases

Mrs C. C.'s sixty trillion bricks were hale, healthy and
sound for seventy years before the toxic substances were able
to attack them, causing her to have what was diagnosed as
'hopeless progressive osteoarthritis'. She was given the usual
large doses of aspirin, and injections to help her pains. But
none of her doctors attempted to look for the cause of the
disease. Consequently the poisons that originally caused her
condition, together with the large doses of aspirin, without
doubt continued more and more to attack her joint bricks,
causing her to be confined to a wheelchair.

When Mrs C. followed my diet, she had an almost
immediate recovery, and she is now in good health. Even at
seventy-five years of age, when the poisons were removed,
her trillions of bricks were able to regenerate, so that Mrs C.
was able to have 'flashes of strength' and to be 'full of youthful energy'.

In the second case, Mr P. E. was diagnosed as having
rheumatoid arthritis. His several doctors had followed the
usual procedure of giving him large doses of aspirin and also
a cortisone derivative. His condition became worse, and
here we have the identical circumstances as Mrs C.'s case.
The original poison plus large doses of aspirin damaged

trillions of the bricks in his body, making it impossible for him to walk. When he followed my diet, these bricks regenerated, and he was relieved of all his pain and discomfort.

These two cases are typical of the many arthritis cases that have had remarkable remissions after being on my diet. Their recovery seems dramatic and almost unbelievable after what they went through with the usual orthodox treatment. To be sure, not all rheumatic disease cases will get dramatic relief merely by following the diet alone, because their cases may be complicated by other diseases. For this reason, I advise everyone who has arthritis to have a complete physical examination periodically.

# 4

# Food allergy and arthritis

Allergy to food has been known for thousands of years. In the year 3000 BC, China's first emperor, Shen Nung, and his physicians observed that some people developed hives, which they called *fung non*, after eating certain types of seafood. They described it as an itching skin disease that produced red blotches or welts and either occurred in local areas of the body or was generalised. Other symptoms associated with the disease were vomiting, diarrhoea, dizziness and difficulty in breathing. As a result Shen Nung decreed that all pregnant women in China must stop eating seafood. He reasoned that the 'poison' that caused *fung non* might cause miscarriages and possibly other disorders.

Egyptians, too, knew of the ailments created by allergy, for the symptoms are chronicled on their tablets and on the walls of their tombs.

And Lucretius, the Roman poet and part-time physician who lived during the first century BC, has been credited with the adage, 'One man's meat is another man's poison.' In the Old Testament dietary restrictions were outlined because through observation and experience certain foods were noted to create physical disorders. But other early doctors were baffled by manifestations of diseases brought on by food – for why should one person be able to eat meat and feel well, while another person becomes ill on the same fare?

## Statistics on allergic diseases today

Authorities say that in the United States there are approximately one hundred million people who have some sort of allergy – to the air that they breathe, which causes sneezing or asthma; to what they eat or drink, which causes stomachaches or diarrhoea, or to things that they touch, which gives them a skin reaction. This is what we call an allergy – a person is allergic to certain substances which somehow make him ill.

American industry loses two hundred million work-days annually because workers are sick with allergy-related diseases; the medical and drug costs are approximately three hundred million dollars yearly. Because of occupational skin disorders another 750,000 people do not report to work. Allergy is the most common chronic disease of childhood. Possibly fifteen million children have allergic problems that should be treated by doctors, but only a third of them receive any medical care.

Allergy can be a serious, crippling and fatal disease in children. It accounts for millions of school days lost annually. Asthma alone causes more deaths in children than any other disease, except tuberculosis. Among American adults it is estimated that there are ten million suffering from asthma – and that there are ten thousand deaths resulting from it yearly.

But the public as a whole has not been very concerned with allergy because compared to other diseases, allergic diseases cause few deaths – they only make life miserable and debilitating. Only people who are afflicted with allergies or have children with allergic diseases are greatly concerned.

Our great achievements in science have only increased allergens – the substances that cause allergic diseases – a hundredfold. For instance, smog, a mixture of fog and pollutants from industrial waste and petrol-driven vehicles, has made cities hazardous to live in. In Los Angeles the atmosphere is so polluted that doctors recommend that the elderly and people with respiratory diseases move out of the city if possible.

Obviously, anything that can help solve the problems of allergy will be of great value, and it is most important to emphasise the science of allergy in the training of our future doctors.

## Allergy and the medical profession

However the science of allergy, like the science of nutrition, is not taught in most medical schools. In fact, a survey of seventy medical schools in the United States indicated that ninety-five per cent of them gave very little, if any, training in the subject of allergy. This is why allergy is sometimes called the stepchild of medicine.

Medical schools today are bacteriologically oriented. As a result, many doctors, when confronted with a disease not related to microbial agents, are puzzled. For example, hospital charts will frequently read: 'migraine headaches, unknown origin'; 'polyneuritis, unknown origin'; 'bursitis, unknown origin'. In my opinion, many such diseases of unknown origin could be allergy-related, and my clinical experience shows that seventy-five per cent of these types of cases respond to dietary measures.

## Specific examples of diseases caused by allergy to food

Dr William Philpott, a research director at the Fuller Memorial Hospital in South Attleboro, Massachusetts, in an article in the San Francisco *Examiner*, said: 'What is now being diagnosed as schizophrenia may in fact be no more than an allergy.' He believes that it is an allergic reaction, resulting in the swelling of the patient's brain, that causes the mental disorder.

Dr Philpott thinks that approximately eighty per cent of mankind suffers from allergic reactions and that the reactions are not always as obvious as when one breaks out in hives after eating strawberries.

The article further stated, 'Dr Philpott said ninety-two per cent of the patients he examined reacted to something. . . . Wheat was the most common irritant, causing reactions in sixty-four per cent; followed by [sweet] corn, fifty-one per cent; and milk, fifty per cent. The average patient reacted to ten things. No patient reacted to just one.'

The distinguished allergist Dr Ben F. Feingold, chief emeritus of the allergy department of the Kaiser Foundation Hospital in San Francisco, in his studies of hyperkinetic children – children with behaviour disturbances and learning difficulties – tells of cases of wall-climbing, head-knocking and uncontrollable impulsiveness. He cites a case of a seven-year-old child who was so aggressive that he would charge at cars while riding on his bicycle. Although many of the children were of normal or high IQ, they had learning difficulties because they manifested such impetuousness that they could not get the words out of their mouths and they were unable to sit still long enough to concentrate on their schoolwork. Dr Feingold found that artificial flavours and colours, some vitamins, hot dogs and such ordinary foods as apples, peaches, apricots, cucumbers, tomatoes and berries can cause hyperactivity in these children.

When the children were put on a special diet, these conditions cleared up completely. Dr Feingold said, 'Children on medication with behaviour-modifying drugs such as amphetamines, methylphenidates, tranquillisers and anti-depressants were able to discontinue the drugs, even with a history of many years of such therapy.'

Dr Marguerite Stemmerman, a West Virginia specialist at the Owen Institute of Nervous and Mental Disorders, reported a case of a one-year-old child with multiple petit mal seizures. She found they were due to the additive MSG (monosodium glutamate). In three days after MSG was deleted from the child's diet the attacks stopped dramatically, and while on the MSG-free diet the child was free of all seizures. In an experiment one year later, the child was given one-half of a frankfurter containing MSG, and within three hours the seizures of petit mal again recurred. Since then the child has stayed on the MSG-free diet and has enjoyed good health without incident.

In 1972, Dr Jean Mayer, Professor of Nutrition at Harvard University, reported a case of a ten-year-old boy who died from an allergic reaction to eating peanuts.

Recent reports indicate that nearly four thousand people in the United States die from choking to death because of food obstructions every year. These attacks which occur frequently in restaurants, are often mistaken for heart attacks and thus have become known as 'café coronaries'. Without doubt, a large number of these incidents are similar to what happened to the ten-year-old boy. In medical terminology this is called an angioedoema of the larynx, which means asphyxiation due to the swelling of the throat caused by an allergic reaction to food and food additives.

Drs J. A. Rudolph and D. M. Rudolph, both specialists in allergy at the University of Miami School of Medicine, said in their excellent book *Allergies – What They Are and What to Do about Them*: '. . . recent studies have revealed that such illnesses as rheumatic fever, rheumatoid arthritis, schleroderma, dermatomyositis and certain forms of nephritis, anaemias and blood and blood vessel diseases resemble hypersensitivity reactions which have been produced in the laboratory.'

Dr Howard G. Rapaport and Shirley Motter Linde, MS, in *The Complete Allergy Guide*, state: '. . . one patient had no problem with milk when she was a child, but in later life developed severe sensitivity reaction to it. Every day that she drank milk for breakfast, about two hours later she had diarrhoea – two days later the joints of her arms and legs became tender and swollen . . . by watching her diet she has not had any attacks.'

They report another case of a '. . . . woman who had suffered with asthma for twenty-eight years. Nothing seemed to help . . . it was discovered that she was sensitive to milk. A quarter of a century of misery from asthma was ended as soon as she eliminated milk and milk products from her diet.'

### Evidence of diseases caused by food allergy largely ignored

Millions of people suffer from allergic diseases which create alarming physical and mental disabilities. Research in various fields has suggested that the combination of the relative abundance of food in the Western world and the poor eating habits of its populations is causing a spectrum of diseases. Improper nutritional habits have either contributed to or caused heart diseases, kidney disorders, lung ailments, hypertension, diabetes, obesity, strokes and even mental disorders.

The medical profession can no longer afford to neglect the study of allergy and nutrition. There is ever-increasing clinical evidence to support the necessity of understanding their effects on the human body.

## Rheumatic diseases caused by allergy

Allergists are in fact the only group of physicians who have suggested that the cause of rheumatic diseases is allergy. Their theory is that rheumatoid arthritis is caused by a form of allergy called auto-immunity, a phenomenon in which the body's defence system goes awry, and turns against the body's own tissues. Ordinarily the defence system only manufactures antibodies against foreign substances such as disease germs, viruses and certain chemicals. The body has a built-in mechanism to prevent its defence system from attacking its own tissues.

According to *The Complete Allergy Guide*, 'No one really knows what brings about the appearance of these self-destroying antibodies known as auto-antibodies. Scientists don't know whether it is a result of ageing, injury, the action of enzymes or even the action of viruses or bacteria.

'The auto-immune processes occur in a wide variety of places; in the gastro-intestinal tract, in the muscles, the joints, the blood, the nervous system, the glands, the eyes.

'Every year physicians attribute more and more diseases to the auto-immune reactions. They include arthritis . . . and systemic lupus erythematosus.'

Let me take you to my Fantasyland once more to try to explain auto-immunity in a different way.

## City of Fantasia

In this city there is a huge manufacturing plant that produces solid-gold replicas of a human body. A force of 20,000 workers is employed on a twenty-four-hour basis, for there is a great demand for this unusual product throughout the world.

To protect this large complex the management imported 2,000 giant panda bears from Tibet. These beautiful animals are world-renowned for their ability to guard large buildings. Their intelligence equals that of a human being, and in addition, they have an unfailing instinct that enables them to distinguish between employees and outsiders, even at night. They never make a mistake between friend or foe.

However, these giant panda bears have one quirk. When they attack anyone, they bite only their joints – the ankles, knees, hips, elbows and shoulders.

For many years there were no burglaries because everyone was aware that these giant panda guards were on duty. Through lack of excitement and because they were well-fed – always in a royal manner with the Western well-balanced diet – the animals soon became fat and lazy. Then for no apparent reason, a group of them started to attack many of the employees of the plant just as if they were outsiders. These pandas were immediately isolated, and local doctors tried to treat them, but to no avail. Finally, famous specialists from all over the world were called in.

It is said that fifteen million dollars a year was spent in trying to find the cause of what they called the auto-immune disease that made the giant pandas lose their fine instinct to differentiate between employees and outsiders. In the meantime, the only medication recommended by the famous specialists was large doses of aspirin. For those who did not respond to the aspirin, stronger medications such as Buta-zolidin, Indocid, antimalarial drugs and cortisone were used. Many of the panda bears were also given injections – not the ordinary kind, but gold shots. For the few animals that did not respond to any of the above treatments, cyto-toxic drugs (used in the treatment of cancer) were administered. All these drugs were used to treat the symptoms of the panda disease, but they did not cure it.

The scientists' failure to find the cause of the disease after spending so much time and money created much dissatisfaction. Some critics contended that because the scientists were trained to believe that all panda diseases were caused by bacteria or viruses, they had spent all their research money in that direction – and they had produced no results. Yet there was overwhelming evidence that panda diseases could also be caused by nutritional factors. Angered by this criticism the specialists retaliated by making this blanket statement: 'The relationship between diet and panda disease has been thoroughly and scientifically studied. The simple proven fact is: no food has anything to do with causing panda disease and no food is effective in treating or curing it.'

One critic, out of curiosity, went to the famous University of California medical library and searched through twenty years of the *Index Medicus* but could not find a single written scientific document to prove that statement.

Another critic theorised that since these beautiful animals were from Tibet, feeding them the luxurious American well-balanced diet 'poisoned' the area of their brains that control their instinct, thus causing the panda disease.

The evidence to support this was in Dr Feingold's experiments with hyperkinetic children; Dr Stemmerman's MSG-free diet for the one-year-old child with petit mal seizures, and the work of Dr Philpott, who believed that allergy to foods caused mental disorders.

But the great scientists continued to look for that mysterious virus. And this, in effect, is the situation today in the city of Fantasia.

### Food allergens as the cause of arthritis – my hypothesis

I want to repeat here what Dr Howard G. Rapaport said: 'No one really knows what brings about the appearance of these self-destroying antibodies known as auto-antibodies. Scientists don't know whether it is a result of ageing, injury, the action of enzymes or even the action of viruses or bacteria.'

In other words, the key question to this whole puzzle is: what *triggers* the whole reaction, or what is the *inciting agent* that starts the entire process of antibodies attacking their own tissues? (Or what caused the panda bears to lose their instinct to differentiate between employees and outsiders and start biting the employees?)

Most rheumatologists still believe that a virus started the whole event and then disappeared. They have spent years in search of that mysterious parasite, but up to this moment none has been discovered.

My hypothesis as to the cause of arthritis is that the *inciting factors* are food allergens – and food allergens, in my estimation, may be considered a 'poison'. Think again of the definition in *Dorland's Medical Dictionary*: 'poison – any substance which when ingested, or developed within the body in relatively small amounts, by its chemical action may cause damage to structure or disturbance of function.'

In the next few pages I want to give some more of my clinical cases to support my contention – and I'll leave the results for you to evaluate. Again, these cases are not given in the usual formal manner. Each of them was tape-recorded, so the patients could tell their stories as they wished.

NAME: Mr I. Z.
AGE: 71
RESIDENCE: California
OCCUPATION: Jewellery salesman
DIAGNOSIS: Osteoarthritis of the spine
DURATION: Twenty-one years
FIRST VISIT: 19 April 1973
PREVIOUS MEDICATION: Aspirin, Indocid, Butazolidin, steroids
INTERVIEWED: 8 August 1974

'It was July 1952, and I was walking down the street, when I had a strong pain in my ribs. It extended from my back around to my chest. I took a few steps and then rested on a fire hydrant for about twenty minutes. When I felt better, I walked back to my jewellery store, which was about a block away. Every time I put my foot down it felt like a shock. It was very painful. The pain went from my foot straight up to my chest. At that time I was fifty years old.

'I called the local Medical Association, and I asked them to help me. They gave me five or six doctors' names. I picked one out and called him. The first thing he asked me over the phone was if I had the money to pay for the office visit. That made me mad. So I hung up and called another doctor. The second doctor sent me to a hospital for X-rays, mylograms and all kinds of examinations. He gave me a rainbow of pills to take and lots of shots. Nothing happened. I still had the pains. After two months of this kind of treatment the doctor wanted to give me more of the same, so I walked out.

'I travel a lot up and down the Coast because I am a jewellery salesman. Whenever one of my friends in various towns recommended his doctor, I would go to him to see if I could get some relief from all my pain. I had also been to all kinds of physiotherapists. They gave me hot baths, cold baths, hot sand on my back and shoulders. I would get relief for a few hours and then the pain would come back again. In other words, I was getting no results – I felt I was throwing my money away.

'I decided to go to the Mayo Clinic because my sister had been there and had liked it. So I went there with my problems and spent a week. They said that I had osteoarthritis, a kind of disease that there is no cure for. I was very discouraged, but I had to go from one doctor to another trying to get relief from the pains that I had. I finally went to the Veterans Hospital. I was there six times. They also told me that there was no cure for my kind of back trouble. All they gave me was pain tablets.'

[*The case history of Mr I. Z. exemplifies the 'treatment mentality' of most of today's doctors. 'Osteoarthritis is tantamount to instant old age. We can't do anything about the process of ageing, so just take aspirin for the rest of your*

*golden days.' I started him on the diet and gradually had him
cut down on the medication he was taking.*]

'For the first couple of months, I did not seem to get results,
but the pains were disappearing gradually. Then, after six
months, I threw away all the coloured pills that I had been
getting from all the other doctors. I am not taking any tablets
at all now. In fact, about a year ago, I bought some arthritis
pain tablets, and I still have seventy-five of the one hundred
tablets. My wife takes one once in awhile. But I do not take
them any more.

'I work in the garden, I walk and ride in my car without
any pain. In fact, I just came back from Miami last week. I
am entirely a different person now. I weighed 12¼ stone a
year ago and now I weigh only 11. I feel like a young man. I
feel like I had two lives – one that I had with pains for twenty
years, and one that I have now without pain.'

[*Mr I. Z. responded to my treatment programme so well that
he recently returned from an exploration trip to the Antarctic
to study the sex life of the penguins.*]

NAME: Mrs P. S.
AGE: 28
RESIDENCE: Colorado
OCCUPATION: Housewife
DIAGNOSIS: Rheumatoid arthritis
DURATION: Two and a half years
PREVIOUS MEDICATION: 20 aspirin a day, prednisone
    orally, Indocid, Butazolidin alka, Naproxen
FIRST VISIT: 16 August 1974
INTERVIEWED: 16 August 1974

'About two and a half years ago, a month after the birth of
my child, I found myself extremely fatigued. I began to feel
stiffness and pain in my joints, especially in the morning. At
first I thought it was simply the after effects of my pregnancy.
However, soon my joints started to swell, first in my fingers,

then in my wrists and shoulders and finally down to my knees. After completing a series of laboratory tests and X-ray examinations, the doctors told me that the laboratory tests showed that I had rheumatoid arthritis. I was seriously ill for a whole year. I could not bathe myself, or dress myself, or hold my new baby. I could hardly walk.

'I was taking twenty aspirin a day, and also, subsequently, cortisone, Indocid, and Butazolidin alka by mouth. The medicine also made me very ill. I had been taking gold shots too. But nothing seemed to help me, and I got worse and worse. Both of my knees became terribly inflamed and swollen. They became about twice the size of normal knees, and naturally, I could not walk at all then.

'The rheumatologist said that if I did not get better I would have to have them drained. That was what I should expect from the disease rheumatoid arthritis. The doctor made an appointment for me with the hospital to have the knees drained in two weeks.

'In the meantime, I found *The Arthritic's Cookbook*. I went on the diet. When I went back to the rheumatologist in two weeks, my knees were back down to normal size. He could not believe this at all. He said that he had not seen anything like this in his life.'

[*This case is almost a classical textbook picture of rheumatoid arthritis. The American Rheumatism Association has developed clinical criteria for the diagnosis of this disease. The patient had morning stiffness and pain at the beginning of her illness. And in addition, there was swelling in the joints of her hands, wrists and shoulders on both sides. Later both knees became swollen with fluid which her doctor planned to drain. These signs and symptoms are almost exactly as listed in the clinical criteria. Her doctor's laboratory tests confirmed the diagnosis. In addition this disease affects women three times more frequently than men, and the age bracket is usually young adults under the age of forty.*

*The patient was given the usual treatment by her doctors, which began with large doses of aspirin and subsequently Indocid, Butazolidin alka and cortisone. Because she did not respond well with oral medication, she was also given gold therapy.*

*The patient came into my office on 16 August 1974 for one consultation. Since she had already decreased the amount of drug medication herself after her relief by adhering to the Dong Diet, I advised her to continue the Naproxen and one prednisone a day. Naproxen is used mainly as a drug designed to relieve both pain and inflammation. Its side effects are said to be less than those of aspirin.*]

'I do not take any more aspirin. I do not take anything now but a Naproxen and one prednisone a day.

'I do not have any pains any more, and just a little stiffness once in a while. I am not tired any more during the day like I used to be.'

NAME: Mrs L. De W.
AGE: 67
RESIDENCE: California
OCCUPATION: Retired secretary
DIAGNOSIS: Rheumatoid arthritis
DURATION: 28 years
PREVIOUS MEDICATION: 16 aspirin a day, Darvon twice a day, gold therapy, steroid injections when pain is severe, Butazolidin and Butazolidin alka once a day
FIRST VISIT: 31 January 1974
INTERVIEWED: 31 January 1974

'I have had rheumatoid arthritis since I was thirty-nine years old. By taking large doses of aspirin and gold shots, I had been able to work until I was sixty-four. Then I retired. I had been taking gold shots, sixteen aspirins a day, Darvon twice a day, Butazolidin once a day, and if the pain became too severe, I would take a cortisone shot. I had also been taking Valium in order to sleep.

'My condition had become so bad that I ached in every part of my body, but especially in my thumbs. I also had spurs on my feet and found it difficult to stand for any length of time.

'I heard about *The Arthritic's Cookbook* and purchased a copy. When I went to see my doctor about four months ago, I asked him if he knew about the diet. I had brought my copy of the book to his office for him to see. He said, "Oh, I know about the diet, and I have read the book. My wife bought it. I don't think it would help you, but you can try it."

'Now, three and a half months later, I can drive my car. I can hold a pen and write again. I can dance and I am full of pep. I feel great all over. I can take baths now, because I can lower myself into the tub, where I was not able to before. I could not dress myself, or comb my own hair, or even turn the doorknob to get in or out of a room. Now I can do all those things. I could not wash my neck because I could not get my hands and arms around to do this. . . . I am so happy to be able to do these things now.

'I had a thyroid nodule that interfered with my swallowing once in a while; now this has disappeared. My doctor is amazed with my progress. The last time that he examined me he said that I was in better health now than I have been since I first came to see him. I asked him if I should continue on with Dr Dong's Diet, and he said, "By all means, do not go off it at all!" '

NAME: Mrs N. C.
AGE: 63
RESIDENCE: Idaho
OCCUPATION: Housewife
DIAGNOSIS: Rheumatoid arthritis with concomitant osteo-
arthritis
DURATION: 4 years
PREVIOUS MEDICATION: Aspirin, Indocid, steroid in-
jections, steroids orally
FIRST VISIT: 12 August 1974
INTERVIEWED: 16 August 1974

'I have had arthritis for the past four years. It started in my right elbow and migrated down to both knees in 1972. The right knee was bad, and became increasingly worse. It was so severe that I could hardly walk. I first went to a hospital.

After a series of examinations, the doctor stated that I had rheumatoid arthritis and that nothing could be done for me. He suggested that I take aspirin for the pains.

'Then I went to see another specialist. All last summer both of my knees were so swollen that I had to put hot packs on them, even during the worst heat of the summer. I could not get up from my bed unless I put these hot packs on my knees.

'After another series of examinations, this new doctor said that I had osteoarthritis, so he gave me several shots of cortisone in the knees. The injections gave me a little relief from the pain, but the swelling did not go down at all.

'Dr Dong's book was recommended to me by a friend. I was in the hospital at the time, and when I went home, I followed the diet quite closely. Although I disliked fish before I began the diet, I ate it. Doing without dairy products didn't bother me either, because it was worth it to get better. I began to feel a lot better and improved continuously. I lost some of the stiffness, and the swelling in both my knees began to go down. I weighed about $11\frac{1}{2}$ stone, and I lost a stone on the diet. This helped me quite a bit.

'The best thing was that I had lots of steps in my home, and I could not manage them before. Now I go up and down with no trouble.'

NAME: Mrs B. R.
AGE: 70
RESIDENCE: California
OCCUPATION: Retired employee of telephone company
DIAGNOSIS: Rheumatoid arthritis, generalised, involving both hands, elbows, shoulders, knees and both feet
DURATION: 4 years
PREVIOUS MEDICATION: Prednisone, Indocid, aspirins
FIRST VISIT: 30 November 1972
INTERVIEWED: 13 August 1974

'In 1969 I retired from the telephone company. The first symptoms of my arthritis started in my hands a few months before I retired. I was able to use the computer and the other office equipment, but my hands would pain me on and off. During the next two years the disease got worse and spread to other parts of my body. I live on the second floor of an apartment building, and it was very hard to get up the stairs and down them again. I had to grasp the sides of the banister to pull myself up. The doctor was giving me aspirin at first, and added Indocid later on. Then he gave me prednisone when the pain persisted and I was not able to stand it any more. All these medicines did not seem to help me very much. They relieved me at times, when I took large doses. I had pains all day long and at night I would have to get out of bed and sit in a chair when the pains in my shoulders were bad. I was only able to walk one or two blocks before the pains became too severe to continue on. I could not drive my car, because every time I would have to step on the brakes, I could barely stand the pains. If this condition had continued any longer I know that I would have had to enter a convalescent home. I would have lost my independence.'

[*Mrs B R. was put on the Dong Diet. Her medication was continued as prescribed by her previous doctor, but was gradually reduced as she improved. Now the patient takes an occasional Indocid capsule or prednisone whenever she shows any symptoms of pains. She has been asked to return for a check-up examination in six months.*]

'Now I am able to walk up and down the stairs in my apartment building without pains. I have been able to sleep all night lying down instead of sitting up in a chair. I have just returned from a Caribbean cruise and have a few pains now. Perhaps something in the vacation diet has bothered me; but I am seventy years old now and I expect a few pains now and then. However, I can drive my car now and do my own housework. I just cannot believe that I am feeling this well.'

There is a great deal of basic research going on in the fields of allergy and nutrition. The mystifying question is why some people develop allergies while others do not. The chemical warfare between the invading foreign bodies and the defence system of the individual – with the resulting reaction known as allergy – is still unclear to medical scientists.

As practising doctors with multitudes of patients seeking relief from the agonies and pains of arthritis, we must not wait for laboratory scientists to find a definitive cure for the disease if there are other means of giving relief and effecting remissions.

My hypothesis, that rheumatic diseases are caused by chemical poisoning and allergy to foods, has accomplished these goals. As you can see from the typical cases cited earlier on, treatments with the Dong Diet are not only effective but also dramatic. But let me repeat here again that I am not a research scientist. To discover the biochemical facts about the relation of diet to rheumatic diseases requires rigorous and painstaking research of a kind that I have neither the training nor the time to perform.

### What is the Dong Diet?

The diet that I recommend is a basic one. It includes the fundamentals of protein, vitamins, minerals and carbohydrates. However, there are restrictions on certain kinds of foods, which are detailed in the second section of this book.

Two such restrictions are on milk and milk products and fruit and fruit juices. From my years of clinical experience, and after trial and error, I have found that these categories of edibles, recommended by the proponents of the so-called well-balanced Western diet, are, in fact, deleterious to arthritic patients.

Fruits and fruit juices have become an obsession, particularly with the American public, and millions of Americans faithfully drink juice every morning. This merely demonstrates how advertising can brainwash people.

But plenty of other people survive quite well without their glass of 'Florida sunshine' every morning.

Dr Feingold reports that the elimination of certain foods, plus a diet free of artificial colourings and flavourings, can, in a matter of a few days, restore a hyperkinetic child's behaviour back to normal. He said, 'You can reproduce the symptoms at will, *turn them on or off*, that is the fantastic part.'

In my clinical experience, I, too, have found it possible to turn symptoms on and off – 'the tap effect' – by controlling patients' diets. Those patients who eat fruit and drink milk will soon manifest symptoms of arthritis. When those items are removed from their diet, the symptoms disappear.

It is extremely important to understand that once someone goes on my diet, he or she must stay on it for the rest of his life. Many people write to me saying that, now that they feel so much better, wouldn't it be all right to once in a while eat just a little fruit or just a little steak? My answer is always no. What is the point of getting rid of the poisons in our bodies if before long we put them right back in? Even at my age and considering the length of time I have been pain-free, if I go off the diet I feel it literally within hours. Recently someone gave my family some beautiful fresh asparagus. I love asparagus but I have discovered that I shouldn't eat it. This time I was very much involved in this book, and in other things, and I forgot and had some for dinner. The next day my elbow was stiff and a little painful. I thought back to what I might have eaten and realised it must have been the asparagus. So, strict adherence to the diet is essential, always, if you want to remain without pain.

My diet is low in saturated fatty acids, has adequate protein, vitamins and minerals, and carbohydrates, with all the necessary nutrients. It is a diet that eliminates all the ingredients such as high fat content in animal proteins that are the cause of many of the degenerative diseases mentioned earlier. One would think that such a diet would be very bland, but the August 1973 issue of *Woman's Day* magazine, said: 'The dishes are simply so delicious, and so suitable for almost any diet, that we offer them as good eating for everyone.'

Beef, lamb and pork are out, but don't let that alarm you. A bulletin issued by the United States Department of the Interior in September 1961 supports the value of fish, a mainstay of my diet, as a substitute for the usual meat proteins in any diet. This bulletin states, 'Fish can be consumed three times daily, due to its nutritional value, and in general is applicable to any diets designed to yield (1) needed biologically valuable trace minerals; (2) high levels of vitamins, especially of the B-complex system; (3) reduction in sodium intake and consequent reduction in body water retention; (4) reduction in hard-fat intake and restoration of fatty acid balance between hard and soft fats; (5) high levels of readily available, biologically complete, easily digestible proteins; and (6) increase in body energy food-intake, with maximum ease of metabolic utilisation.'

To those in the medical world, I have this to say: my dietary concept has given relief to thousands of arthritic victims, so it must have some therapeutic merit and value. At the very least, it should produce among medical scientists of integrity the desire to seek substantiation. In light of the millions who suffer from arthritis, it does not seem right that any possibility of helping them should be rejected out of hand.

I suggest that doctors use my dietary concept as they have been using aspirin, *empirically*, until the mechanism of why it works is substantiated. For the Dong Diet of fish, chicken, vegetables and simple carbohydrates cannot, by any stretch of the imagination, harm any patient.

My dietary approach in the therapy of rheumatic diseases, as suggested in this book, places in doctors' hands a tool of the utmost importance. It is an addition to their specialised knowledge and an indispensable adjunct to their modes of treatment I know that the more creative and secure among them will approach this nutritional and biochemical therapy with an open mind.

# 5

# Arthritis and sexuality

Arthritis need not take the joy out of sex. But, so often it does! As if an arthritic does not have enough trouble, he is often plagued by problems concerning his sexuality. Sexuality is the constitution of an individual in relation to his sexual attitudes and activity.

Can the Dong Diet help arthritics with sexual problems? Yes. After an explanation of the 'facts of life' for an arthritic and his sexual partner, and after the patient stays on the diet, there is usually a remarkable recovery and a rekindling of interest in sexual relations.

### Sexual concerns of the victims of arthritis and their partners

It has been my clinical observation that the primary concern of the healthy partner of an arthritic is that sexual intercourse may weaken or hurt the other person, or cause an exacerbation of the disease. The partner may also be reluctant to have sexual relations with an arthritic because of a fear that arthritis may be infectious.

When I tell the patients and their partners the 'facts of life', I assure them that there is no foundation for the belief that sexual relations will weaken or injure the arthritic or that it will worsen the condition. I tell them that the healthy partner would never become 'infected' with arthritis because of sexual intercourse.

Where it is the woman who is suffering from arthritis, many couples limit their sexual activities for fear of causing a pregnancy. They are afraid that the wife will be unable to care for a child, and they also fear the additional economic burden. Many couples simply do not want children. The trouble is, they are afraid of the contraceptive pills on the market today. Arthritics fear strokes, cancer, phlebitis and other blood dystrophies. The recent controversy in the media has led physicians and patients alike to question the use of the pill. But there are other contraceptive devices available which do not create this problem. The matter is really one for the individuals concerned, their personal physicians and gynaecologists.

There is also the fear that the child will be born an arthritic. However, thousands of children of rheumatoid arthritic patients are born with no evidence of the disease. (This, incidentally, supports my belief that rheumatoid arthritis is *not* caused by any viral or microbial agents.)

Fear of pregnancy should no more keep persons from engaging in sexual intercourse than fear of injury to an arthritic or fear that it may be 'catching'.

## Advice to the lovelorn

My advice to arthritic patients and their partners is to carry on with their sexual activities if at all possible. Sex is a natural psychological and biological function. Arthritics have enough problems without the frustrations, nervous tensions and anxiety neurosis that often accompanies a lack of sexual relations. There are many additional stresses in the lives of an arthritic and his partner, and where sexual frustrations are present, the relationship may suffer seriously, communication becomes more difficult and often virtually impossible.

## Mental and physical adjustments

While there is usually no reason not to engage in sexual activities, there is usually every reason to approach it in a different manner. Use a practical, common-sense approach, and make adjustments as they are called for. The physical limitations of the arthritic must be considered. Couples must find coital positions that are the easiest and most comfortable for the patient and his partner. Remember that in our present society, any position or means of sexual gratification between two consenting adults can be considered normal and proper. There are many books written by doctors and/or specialists on the subject of sexology. I recommend that the reader consults the various works of Masters and Johnson and their associates, and perhaps, *The Joy of Sex*, by Dr Alex Comfort.

In Dr Alfred Kinsey's, *Sexual Behaviour of the Human Female*, he relates, 'Nearly all of the females in the sample recorded that they had most frequently used a coital position in which the male was above while the female lay supine beneath, facing the male . . . this is the traditional position throughout European and American cultures, and to many persons, it may seem to be the only biologically normal position . . . there are many males and some females who are psychologically stimulated by considering the possibilities of the positions which two human bodies can assume in coitus . . . there have been attempts to calculate the mathematic possibilites of the combinations and recombinations of human forms in coital relationships . . .'

Attitude is all important. Old-fashioned notions about 'proper' coital positions must be changed. Inhibitions must be got rid of. Pleasing a sexual partner can be accomplished by consideration for what gratifies him or her, and almost anything goes. Sex is not a mechanical athletic event, for which scores are kept. It is a biological urge and the consequence of a psychological need for closeness with another person.

## The elderly arthritic

One of the tragedies of arthritis is the sharp decline of the desire for sexual contact, due both to psychological and physical factors. Medication that is used to relieve arthritics of their pain, often has tranquillising and sedative effects on elderly arthritics, and depress the libido. Elderly people frequently terminate their sexual activities altogether, because of the absurd idea that sexual relationships may shorten their life expectancy. On the contrary many patients, including the elderly, who follow my dietary and medical regimen experience a revival of psychological and biological functions.

Some of them are surprised that they are able to resume sexual activities again, and have happily returned to my office to inform me of this 'phenomenon'. Here is yet another demonstration of what I previously mentioned as the 'cause–effect–cure' syndrome. (The cells that make up the genital organs regenerate to revive the sexual abilities, because the poison is gone from their bodies.)

Gerontologists and medical scientists feel that we should live to be at least one hundred years, and retain physical as well as mental vigour. Dr Eric Pfeiffer of Duke University has mentioned that couples continue to be sexually active in their seventies, eighties and, in some cases, in their nineties. While a gradual decline is the rule, thirteen per cent of the two hundred and fifty-four men and women volunteers that Dr Pfeiffer studied reported *increasing* sexual activity with advancing age.

### Conclusion

In the last decade sexual attitudes have rapidly undergone revolutionary changes. People are beginning to understand that sex is a basic emotional and psychological necessity for both men and women. Today sexual behaviour and the emotions that surround personal relationships are being discussed openly.

Sexual conventions and prohibitions imposed on our society in the past are responsible for a large number of maladjusted unhappy couples. People constantly consult doctors about sex-related dilemmas. This important biological function should be stripped of all its mysteries and taboos, through proper education.

I hope that this chapter has provided some enlightenment. I have directed you to further information. I hope that I have begun to remove some sexual taboos for arthritics and their sexual partners. Over the years, the Dong Diet and a common-sense approach to sexual relations has worked wonders for my patients and their partners. I hope it does the same for you.

# 6

## Exercise and the arthritic

'Every adult should find time in his daily schedule for some form of physical activity,' says the United States President's Council on Physical Fitness. 'Medical evidence tells us that our hearts, lungs, muscles and even our minds need the effects of regular vigorous exercise.'

The majority of the people in the world seem to get along without special exercise programmes. For the people in the state of Hunza in Pakistan and the Vilcabambians, high in the Andes Mountains, for instance, climbing the terraces daily to plant and harvest their food is exercise enough.

Most Westerners start exercise programmes in kindergarten and many continue on through school and college, but if they enter the world of commerce, only a few of them find time to exercise regularly before or after a day of hard work.

Office workers, in their sedentary jobs, do little exercising until the week-ends. Most manual workers, however, use their muscles in performing their jobs so are constantly exercising. For many housewives, their household chores and gardening constitute sufficient physical activity – although it may not be what the President's Council on Physical Fitness considers 'regular vigorous exercise'.

### What is exercise?

Exercise enthusiasts, who jog for miles, play lively games of tennis and engage in other strenuous physical activities have one concept of exercise. They feel that vigorous physical exertion is beneficial for one's health.

My concept of exercise for the arthritic patient may seem less ambitious; it is the performance of mild physical exertion to correct physical deformities. But before therapeutic exercises can begin, the pain, muscle spasms and joint inflammation must be relieved.

The arthritic's only desire is to be able to get out of bed in the morning, to be able to take a bath, to be able to raise his arms to comb his hair, to be able to get in and out of a chair – and someday to be able to drive his own car again, so that he can be self-reliant. These simple functions of life are the 'exercises' that the arthritic would like to accomplish.

## When can an arthritic start exercising?

My first objective with rheumatic disease patients is to free them of their pain. It has been my clinical experience over a period of years that the Dong Diet, with a moderate amount of proper medication, will usually accomplish this purpose.

As I see each patient recovering gradually from the ravages of this tragic disease, I am reminded of how fortunate I am to have recuperated myself. Just recently, a thirty-year-old former airline hostess, with a four-year history of rheumatoid arthritis, came to my office and exclaimed, 'I've only seen you a few times, but last week I went shopping without my cane.' A seventy-four-year-old golfer, whose arthritis had affected his shoulders, neck and back for several years, told me enthusiastically that he was now able to play nine holes of golf without pain. And a sixty-seven-year-old housewife embraced me with tears in her eyes and said, 'Doctor, I went wading in the Pacific Ocean for the first time in ten years.'

To these patients *exercise* is to be able to accomplish the *simple functions we take for granted*. That such a goal is possible is the reason I awake each morning stimulated and eager to go to my office to meet the new challenges of each 'apparently hopeless' patient. I know that with my treatment methodology I can give a measure of hope, relief and mobility to every new case. This is my elixir of life.

When my patients, or their families, ask me when to start exercising, I tell them that the best way to tell is by the

presence or the absence of pain. It is important to exercise
as soon as the pain decreases, in order to prevent atrophy of
the muscles and immobility of the bones or joints. It is
equally important to stop exercising if there is pain.

### What kind of exercise should the arthritic do?

I suggest that arthritics avoid being spectators. I advise them
to participate in sports as soon as possible. However, I warn
them not to try to be competitive and not to exhaust themselves.

Indoor swimming in a heated pool is particularly beneficial, because the body is suspended in water and the
movements put no undue strain on the joints. The contrac-
tion and stretching of the muscles in the warm water
increases the circulation throughout the body, giving the
patient a feeling of well-being.

Walking in the fresh air is the very best exercise that an
arthritic can do, slowly or briskly, depending upon your
ability and desire. Taking a few deep breaths while walking
increases the oxygen supply to the lungs, so one should
remember to do this intermittently. Most people are not too
far from a museum or gallery. Doing one's walking in this
kind of setting is not only educational and fun but good for
the arthritic as well. If the patient takes an interest in what
he is doing it does not seem like programmed exercise, and
he is more willing to participate.

### Books on exercise

I would think that more books, pamphlets and articles have
been written on exercise than on any other subject, except
perhaps on sex. For those of you who would like to experiment with new and different types of exercise, look for books
on kung fu, yoga or isometrics. Try doing some of the
exercises that are outlined, but use your discretion and do
not exhaust yourself.

## Relevant case histories

The August 1974 issue of the American journal *Medical Opinion* featured on its cover a picture of a cane, a handful of capsules, some pills and a stack of hospital bills and cancelled cheques. The caption was: 'Low-Back Pain Syndrome, He's Crippled by Pain, Hooked on Medication, Burdened by Bills.'

This rather graphic description accurately fits most of my patients who have gone through years of orthodox treatment programmes. The mere mention of exercise or any physical exertion terrifies most of them. But by adhering strictly to my dietary and medical plans, not only are they able to exercise, they have returned to gainful work as well.

The following case histories are relevant to this discussion:

NAME: Mr W. V.
AGE: 67
RESIDENCE: California
OCCUPATION: Retired municipal employee
DIAGNOSIS: Rheumatoid arthritis
DURATION: Six years
PREVIOUS MEDICATION: Aspirin, Indocid, gold therapy
FIRST VISIT: 4 June 1973
INTERVIEWED: 6 May 1974

'In 1968 I was told that I had arthritis. The doctor that I went to gave me all kinds of examinations and finally said that I had rheumatoid arthritis. It began in both my hands and went down to my knees and legs on both sides.

'I was treated by my last specialist for five years. He gave me gold shots, aspirin and everything that is usually used for this disease. Still my condition worsened every year. Both of my hands were crippled and I could hardly use them. By 1973 I was on crutches and could hardly walk – I was dragging one leg around and could not bend my knees.'

*[The patient was started on the diet and I told him to have his*

*wife call me so I could give her instructions on how to cook for him.*]

'I feel fine now. I walk four or five miles without any trouble. I go to my front garden and dig the ground and plant things. I do not have any problems at all. I do all kinds of work around the house, and just last month I remodelled the whole kitchen. I stained the wood, put on cabinet doors, did all the plumbing and electrical work myself – getting up and down from the floor without any trouble. Nothing, nothing hurts me!

'The only time I have any aches is when I overwork and stay in the garden too long. Then I go in to have my lunch and take a siesta.'

NAME: Mrs I. D.
AGE: 58
RESIDENCE: California
OCCUPATION: Housewife
DIAGNOSIS: Rheumatoid arthritis
DURATION: Since the age of twelve
PREVIOUS MEDICATION: Aspirin, steroids, 'and every new kind of medicine that they could give me'
FIRST VISIT: 7 March 1974
INTERVIEWED: 6 December 1974

'I have had rheumatoid arthritis for many years. The pains were terrible. I could not walk, could not sleep, and my knees, shoulders, hands, neck, and all over my body ached until it was almost unbearable. Pains in my hands were so bad that I would just sit there and cry. Every time I telephoned my doctor to complain, he would just tell me to increase the aspirin. Even then the pains were not alleviated and I would take a few more in the hopes of relief. My case was diagnosed by an specialist as rheumatoid arthritis. Periodically I would have attacks when I would have to go back on crutches and stay in bed completely.'

[*Mrs I. D. had begun the diet on her own after her daughter-in-law read about my book.*]

'The pains started to let up in about a week or two, after I had begun the diet. I began to walk without pain and was not taking aspirin. Within a month even the stiffness started to leave me. I began to do all my own housework again, and the cooking also.

'When I was very ill it was so painful to get out of my bed to go to the bathroom that I had to be helped. But as I began to get well from the diet, I could feel myself straightening up again – and my husband would say to the children, "Doesn't your mother look wonderful again?"

'Now I am feeling so well that I am going to start taking tennis lessons soon. Yesterday I played tennis with my daughter and rallied back and forth. Every time my son looks at me, he says he cannot believe it is the same mother that was bed-ridden and in such pain.'

NAME: Mrs S. N.
AGE: 62
RESIDENCE: Louisiana
OCCUPATION: Housewife
DIAGNOSIS: Osteoarthritis of the lower spine
DURATION: Three years (with constant pain)
PREVIOUS MEDICATION: Aspirin, Indocid, Darvon
FIRST VISIT: 16 October 1973
INTERVIEWED: 13 November 1974

'I lived with terrible pains in my back for the past few years. I had a bad fall from horseback a few years ago and I never fully recovered from it. It had become increasingly worse to the point that when I sat down in a chair, I could not get out of it at all. In the mornings I could hardly get out of bed. The pains were constant and I almost gave up in despair.

'I had been to various doctors and many specialists for different kinds of treatments, but it had done me no good. Finally I heard about Dr Dong. With his strict diet and treatments, I can now go out and get on one of the cable cars here in San Francisco. I can run up and down the stairs and sit in chairs and be able to get out of them again. I can do all those little everyday things that I could not do before. The same is true for walking. I was not able to walk or to do any exercises before. But now in Belvedere, where I am staying with my cousin, I find myself walking over to the boardwalk and shopping. These are things that I was unable to do before.'

# 7

# Longevity:
# Everyone's goal

If you are wondering what a chapter on longevity is doing in a book about arthritis, you will be surprised to learn that the Dong Diet is not only beneficial for victims of arthritis, but also has longevity as one of its significant rewards.

Dr Ralph Nelson, chief of the Clinical Nutrition Department of the Mayo Clinic, in Minnesota, said at an American Medical Association conference in 1973, '*There will someday be such a thing as a longevity diet.*' He went on to describe a diet that is already here, the diet that I have been recommending for over thirty-five years. Dr Nelson said, 'It will be a diet to which very little or nothing will be added, but from which a lot of things people now customarily eat will be omitted. That the Americans eat too much is hardly news, but what is news to a lot of people is the fact that the vitamins and other supplements, extra proteins and diet additives recommended by food faddists, not only do no good for the average person, they may do a great deal of harm. They are among the items the longevity diet will omit.'

Once it has been researched and established, Dr Nelson feels, the longevity diet will be low in calories and proteins. Today we in the West are over-indulging in these food elements. He said, 'Americans are shortening their life-span by consuming too much protein . . . we do not store excess protein in our bodies, but excrete it in the form of nitrogen. In very common language, the high-protein diet fills our system with garbage that must be treated by the kidneys. Excess protein forces the body to work harder to get rid of that garbage.'

Dr Nelson concluded that 'People who stuff themselves with high-protein and high-calorie foods shorten their lives. Carbohydrate loading can cause heart trouble and swallowing vitamin supplements can be poisonous.'

## What is old age?

When you reach sixty-five, you are supposed to be entering old age. Everything is geared for retirement – arrangements are made for your medical care; businesses large and small request your retirement; you get a pension. You are brainwashed into believing that your contributions to the active world are terminated and that your skills and experiences are no longer needed. Elsewhere in the world, chronological age is of no concern; personal skills, ability and knowledge are appreciated indefinitely; but in Western society they are ignored.

Sydney J. Harris, in one of his philosophical asides, wrote, 'When I hear of men being forced to retire at 65, I think of Kant writing his *Anthropology* at 74; Tintoretto painting his "Paradise" at 74; Verdi composing his opera *Otello* at 74; Goethe completing his *Trilogy of Passion* at 74 – and Titian painting his historic "Battle of Lepanto" at 98.'

Employment should be based on a person's competence and skill, not his age. Forced retirement can seriously impair mental and physical health – the loss of prestige, loss of routine and loss of activity all contribute to the sense of worthlessness. The nation is then forced to support the pensioner and to lose his or her productivity.

## What is longevity?

Longevity, according to the Oxford Dictionary, is simply 'long life'. But scientists are more definite about how long an individual will live. They estimate that all mammals should live five times the number of years it takes their skeleton to mature. Since a dog matures at three years, fifteen years is the normal life of a dog. A human being matures at twenty-five, therefore, humans should really live to be one hundred and twenty-five years of age. By those standards, then, if a person does not live to be at least a hundred years old, with good health, vigour and vitality, then he is depriving himself of many years of happy living.

## What shortens life?

In the eighteenth century the average length of life was thirty-five to forty years. Most deaths at that time were due to infectious diseases – pneumonia, influenza, tuberculosis, enteritis and diphtheria – because of the lack of preventive medicine and sanitation.

Since the discovery of penicillin by Alexander Fleming, and the development of other antibiotics, the death rate from these diseases has been reduced. Now the average life expectancy is considered to be sixty-nine and a half years. So we are still short of the goal by over fifty years. Non-infectious diseases such as heart disease, atherosclerosis, cerebral vascular diseases, cancer, diabetes, hypertension and arthritis prevent us from attaining the goal. And, as I've already discussed, most of these degenerative diseases can be traced to dietary indiscretion.

## What is gerontology?

*Dorland's Medical Dictionary* defines gerontology as 'the scientific study of the problems of ageing in all aspects – clinical, biological, historical and sociological.'

From the beginning of time, man has been both perplexed and intrigued by the processes of ageing. In the Far Eastern cultures, especially in China, this stage of life has been longed for, accepted and venerated. However, in the United States, ageing is both feared and dreaded.

We cannot deal with every phase of this subject here, but let us see what some specialists in gerontology have found in their research.

Many gerontologists and other medical scientists have come to the conclusion that two of the most vital factors in retarding the ageing process are dieting and exercise. This substantiates my own observations and clinical experiences.

An interesting and erudite study on this subject was made by Dr Alexander Leaf, Chief of Medical Services at Massachusetts General Hospital in Boston, who journeyed to 'several places in the world where it is not unusual for people to live to the age of one hundred and still retain their health and vigour. Such pockets of longevity are to found in the Andean area of Ecuador, the Caucasus Mountains of Russia and in the State of Hunza in Pakistan.' Dr Leaf's article, 'Observations of a Peripatetic Gerontologist,' in *Nutrition Today*, September–October 1973, continued, 'During the past two years, I have visited three corners of the world where aged individuals are free of the debilitating diseases that plague our elderly. I had ample opportunity to observe the dietary customs and conclude that they would give solace to our nutritionists, who seem to have reached the conclusion that we must change our eating habits if we are to live longer. If the United States and Canada had the same proportion of people who are a hundred or more years old as one can see in these areas, there'd be nearly two and a half million centenarians in the two countries. As it is there are only some seven thousand people who have passed the century mark.'

He also noted that hard work seems to be another factor that aids in achieving the goal of longevity. 'If someone told me that James Hilton got his inspiration for his book *Lost Horizon* from Hunza, I would believe him. Shangri-la was the home of the ageless who lived in paradise. It was said to be free of tension, which is supposed to play a role in shortening the lives of Western man. The geography of Hunza requires everyone to work hard to eke a living from the sparse terraces. In spite of (or because of) the primitive conditions, one sees an unusual number of vigorous elderly men and women agilely climbing up and down the steep slopes that line the habitable valley of these mountain dwellers.'

In his studies Dr Leaf found that the diets of the Hunza and Vilcabamba people, who live on a very restricted diet, differ from the people in the Caucasus region, who eat everything (but of course not processed foods). He concluded, 'According to what we are now being told about the aetiology of atherosclerosis, one would say that their low calorie diet, rich in unsaturated fats and vegetables and poor in animal fats, dairy products and sucrose, must account for the longevity of the Hunzakuts and Vilcabambians. But, then, if this is so, what about the Georgians? Their dietary habits and longevity, although different, still give some support to the "low animal fat, low cholesterol, low caloric" school of thought.'

Other prominent gerontologists, after years of meticulous research, have demonstrated a definite correlation between diet and longevity. An article in the San Francisco *Examiner* by Peter Fraley stated, 'Research into the ageing process is demonstrating that the human life-span can be stretched as much as thirty years. Dr Leon R. Kass, of the National Academy of Sciences, points out that research into ageing and senescence is a field just entering puberty. He cites recent studies that show ageing to be a process distinct from disease and one that can be retarded by diet and drugs. A classic study done in the early 1930s, showed that rats kept on a near-starvation diet lived twice as long as a control group that ate as much as they liked. Recently, Dr Roy L. Walford of the University of California, Los Angeles, did similar experiments, cutting the diets of rats and mice to a third of the normal calorie intake. He got similar results of increased life-span and a reduction in the tendency to develop cancer. The exact mechanism for this startling finding remains unknown, but there is an indication that it may be due to a strengthening of the body's resistance to disease. However, the reverse is well known and accepted, that overeating and obesity shorten life in a variety of ways.'

Dr Walford's observation is substantiated by our Western society. Insurance company statistics indicate that there are over fifty million overweight people in America alone. At any given time, men or women, if twenty per cent over their ideal weight, have a twenty per cent higher death rate. As the percentage of overweight goes up, the death rate also increases. People who are thirty to forty per cent above normal weight have a fifty per cent greater chance of dying than those of normal weight.

The Metropolitan Life Insurance Company stated in its bulletin *Overweight – Its Prevention and Significance*, 'Studies were made of a group of men twenty per cent or more over-weight and another group of average-weight men with various diseases. The death rate in the over-weight group was forty per cent higher than in the average-weight group, in those persons with heart and circulatory disorders. In those with cerebral haemorrhage and other vascular disorders, the death rate was fifty per cent higher in the over-weight group than in the average-weight group. In nephritis, seventy-five per cent higher. The death rate in over-weight diabetics was especially high – more than twice that (one hundred and thirty-three per cent) of the average-weight diabetic.'

From this we can only conclude that the way to stop the process of ageing and to build up resistance against all diseases is to control our over-weight problems.

Dr Joseph P. Hrachovec, a University of Southern California gerontologist, agrees. In his well-documented book on anti-ageing, *Keeping Younger and Living Longer*, he wrote that it is entirely possible for people to live past the ages of seventy, eighty and even a hundred years and still be able to enjoy active, healthy lives. People reduce their chances for a longer life, bring on diseases and make the body wear out too quickly by making three mistakes: (1) by eating im-properly, (2) by not exercising and (3) by not being able to relax.

Dr Bernard Strehler, University of California professor of biology, stated that '. . . man can find means to increase his life-span by fifteen to thirty years. For example, animal experiments have shown that the effects of dietary restriction alone can increase the life-span – increasing longevity cannot be brought about without increasing the quality of old people's health. With good health, people in the sixty-five to eighty-five bracket might well remain employed and not become a burden . . . postponement of physical and mental senescence will mean that a person of sixty would have the outlook of a [present-day] person of fifty; the person of seventy, the outlook of a person of fifty-six; and a person of ninety, the outlook of a person of seventy. There would be new opportunities for self-development that a period of forty to fifty years of healthy and vigorous life would offer to mothers following child rearing and to fathers for further training and work.'

Although all these authorities criticise the Western diet, none has specific recipes to correct the dietary indiscretions. I hope this book will help fill that gap.

## Effects of the Dong Diet

The following clinical cases show the role the Dong Diet can play in attaining the goal of longevity:

Mrs R. W. of California was previously mentioned in *The Arthritic's Cookbook*. In 1972 she was Miss R. H., aged seventy-three, who hobbled into my office on a cane for consultation. Her knees, hands and ankles were badly affected with osteoarthritis. Miss R. H. weighed twelve stone at her first examination, and she was taking sixteen aspirin daily. The aspirin were immediately stopped, and she was told to adhere to a stringent diet of fish and vegetables (excluding rice, bread and potatoes until her weight was reduced). Within one month, Miss R. H. weighed ten stone and had thrown her cane away. She was married about a year later.

Last week, sitting across from me at my desk, she looked more like a happy housewife in her late fifties than a woman of seventy-seven. She maintains her weight between ten and eleven stone. She has had no recurrence of her 'crippling arthritis'. On examination, her blood pressure was 145/86; tests of the heart, lungs and other physical findings were all within normal limits. Mrs R. W.'s biochemical blood test last year was also good, and I expect the results from this year's test to be the same – she appears to be in excellent health. She does her own housework and walks up and down the stairs of her two-storey house without effort.

Last year she flew to Denver, Colorado, to attend a class reunion. Her married life has been a 'very happy one'. Mrs R. W. is a fine example of what the Dong Diet can do to prevent arthritis and to increase longevity.

Mrs G. H., aged seventy-four, of Washington, DC, came to me for treatment of her osteoarthritis. It was necessary for her to use a cane to get about, but her hands were so badly deformed she could barely hold it. Mrs G. H. was treated in my office for six weeks – resulting in a remarkable recovery.

Upon returning home to Washington, the patient was able to walk without the use of her cane. She had lost a stone, and most of her friends could not believe she was the same woman. Once while she was shopping at a local market, Mrs G. H. noticed a couple of women whispering about her in one of the aisles. One of them came up to her and asked, 'Are you Mrs H.? What happened to you? You look so young and different – and you are not using your cane. We could not believe it was you!'

Mrs G. H. told me that one of the most rewarding things that has happened to her is her ability to work around the house. Just before she came out to visit me again this year, she was able to turn the mattress of her bed over completely by herself; before her treatments in my office she could hardly make her own bed without assistance.

Mr P. L., aged ninety-six, an osteoarthritis case, has been a patient for many years. One morning he was found unconscious in his hotel room, and I put him in the hospital. He had a severe upper respiratory infection that developed into pneumonia. After ten days in the hospital he was sent home to rest. Soon after, Mr P. L. appeared in my office in his usual happy and cheerful manner, none the worse for his critical illness. He is a well-dressed man without the appearance of most aged bachelors, whose clothes are often stained and unkempt.

I was so proud of his recovery from both pneumonia and osteoarthritis that I accompanied him out to the waiting room to show him off to some of my other patients. I briefly related his history and mentioned that Mr P. L. was ninety-four years of age. He immediately corrected me: 'Dr Dong, I'm ninety-six.'

The above clinical cases demonstrate the effectiveness of a proper diet. These people have become independent, self-sufficient, productive citizens again. There are millions throughout the world who could obtain the same results if they would pay attention to their diet.

## In retrospect

While writing this chapter on longevity, it occurred to me that I myself have long since passed the 'mandatory retirement age'. I have never given it much thought. In the midst of a reasonably full and active life I have not had time for reflection or retrospection. I still play golf, work in my office and carry on community projects with the same zest and enthusiasm. My living schedule has not changed much in the past thirty-five years, except for the added responsibility of writing this book.

A short time ago, my old class at the Stanford University Medical School, the class of 1931, had a reunion. Only seven members came to the meeting. On investigation I found that twenty out of a class of forty-nine were already dead. Only a few classmates are still practising medicine, and only on a part-time basis. If I had not changed my nutritional habits long ago I am certain that I would have been listed among the deceased in the vital statistics of my class, instead of carrying on a full programme of my life's work.

Statistics show that in the United States the high-earning social groups have a higher death rate. Physicians and surgeons in the prime of life lead the parade to the cemetery, followed by lawyers, judges and business executives – and the lowest death rates are among labourers and farmers. This high death rate among the highly skilled is not only a personal loss to families and friends, but also a great loss to the nation.

The science of gerontology has exposed some of the secrets of the process of ageing. The outstanding factors are proper diet and exercise. Only a little discipline on anyone's part is required to carry out a longevity programme that will enable him or her to continue to contribute fully to society right up to the end – and that end should not come before you are a hundred years old.

# 8

# Acupuncture:
## its role in my treatment of arthritis

In 1971 the American President visited China, parting the Bamboo Curtain for the first time in twenty-five years to give us a fascinating glimpse of the sleeping giant. Things of Chinese origin suddenly became of intense general interest.

Groups of prominent physicians, surgeons and medical scientists were invited by the Chinese Medical Association to observe at first hand the health-care systems of China and to exchange ideas with their doctors. The majority were astounded at China's medical progress.

The most controversial medical technique has been the use of acupuncture for the treatment of diseases and especially in the field of anaesthesia. Because of stories that were circulated about 'miracle cures' and the use of acupuncture in major operations, there was pressure on the conservative medical establishment to investigate acupuncture and perhaps adopt it. Today, research programmes on acupuncture are being carried out in American medical schools, and in all parts of the West the first few practitioners are tentatively trying it out.

### History of acupuncture

The earliest known use of acupuncture dates back some four to five thousand years ago, in China. Therefore, much of its origin is veiled in legend. One of the most popular versions of its discovery tells how early Chinese warriors, pierced by arrows during battle, reported the relief of old pains in parts of the body far removed from the arrows' points of entry. The ancient Chinese physicians mapped these acupuncture points on the body to relieve pain and disease. Thus, through the centuries, acupuncture became folk medicine. It was widely used wherever Chinese people congregated.

## My encounters with acupuncture

Eventually, acupuncture needles were made of gold and silver, not only so they would be rust-proof, but also because of the supernatural powers that have always been attributed to these metals throughout the world. (Even today, educated and rational people wear copper bracelets, hoping they will prevent or cure arthritis.) The needles, therefore, were made by goldsmiths, and this is where the saga of the Dong family in America began.

In 1873, my father finished his apprenticeship as a goldsmith in Canton. This ambitious lad of nineteen had been inspired by the glowing tales of California, whose streets were supposedly paved with gold. He borrowed twenty dollars and bought a passage to San Francisco on one of the clipper ships of that era. His ambition was to pick up enough gold to return home to China to practise his new profession. As my father stepped off the gang-plank in San Francisco, he encountered his first anti-Chinese demonstrations. Because the economic boom had come to an end, crowds of hoodlums were trying to prevent Chinese people from coming to America. They feared the immigrants might take the few jobs that were available at that time.

My father finally settled in the Salinas Valley, where he practised his profession of goldsmith among the many Chinese located in that area. He not only made acupuncture needles for the Chinese physicians, but also learned the art of acupuncture.

I recall my first encounter with acupuncture, when I was about eight or nine years old. I remember seeing my dad giving treatments to people. He later became a successful merchant and gave up his other professions of goldsmith and acupuncturist.

My second encounter with acupuncture occurred when I graduated from medical school in 1931. I started my practice of medicine in the heart of San Francisco's celebrated Chinatown. There were at that time about ten thousand Chinese people there, descendants of those who had come to America in the Gold Rush days. Six Western-trained doctors of Chinese origin practised in the community, in competition with approximately a hundred herbalists and acupuncturists. We doctors had a difficult time introducing Western medical concepts to our Chinese patients, who were unusually eclectic. Sometimes they would use medicine that we prescribed, and at other times they would return to herbal medicine and acupuncture for their various disorders.

I was often irritated and frustrated by the suspicious and ambivalent attitudes of my Chinese patients. In retrospect, I can understand their thinking process: if one medical method fails to cure, why not try another? I am embarrassed to think that I was so arrogant and intolerant of other methodologies.

During the next two decades I was constantly in contact with traditional Chinese medicine and acupuncture. Many of my friends and patients told stories of people who had been treated by conventional medical procedures for various chronic ailments without success, and then had been cured by acupuncture in a short time. Since I had been thoroughly indoctrinated with scientific medicine, I continued to scoff at such ancient modes of treatment. I theorised, like many of my Western colleagues, that any improvement by acupuncture was a matter of psychology, mesmerism, hypnotism or the result of a placebo effect.

My third encounter with acupuncture was in 1960. One of my golfing companions is a Far Eastern industrial tycoon. His secret ambition in life is to beat me at golf. He regularly spends about two months a year in the United States trying to accomplish this feat, keeping me constantly supplied with golf balls. During one of his strenuous drives on the golf course, he injured his back and shoulders. An acute condition of this kind could be due to any number of causes, and for diagnosis he was referred to the best specialist in

San Francisco. After two months of conventional treatment and physiotherapy, he still could not swing a golf club. In fact, his condition was getting worse. The diagnosis of his problem was osteoarthritis and lumbar intervertebral disc syndrome. Because of his 'advanced' age and lack of response to the treatments, the prognosis was a grave one. He was told that he might never be able to play golf again. I had visions of losing not only a golfing pal, but also my source of free golf balls.

Due to the urgency of business, the industrialist had to go back to the Far East. The next summer, when he returned, he was able to swing his clubs better than before. He told me that after going home he had been treated by a master acupuncturist, and in a matter of a few weeks he was playing golf again. In fact his game had improved to the point where he could play me on even terms. When his two-month visit was up he insisted that I go back with him to the Far East to investigate acupuncture more thoroughly.

All the threads of my experiences were beginning to come together with the result that I began to have a new and less biased opinion of acupuncture.

My wife and I went to Taipei for a three-week vacation. In fact I stayed several months, not only in Taipei but also in Japan and Hong Kong, studying the principles and techniques of acupuncture. I was amazed at the many complicated cases of whiplash, low-back syndrome, 'frozen shoulder', various types of arthritis and other painful conditions that were relieved by acupuncture, especially since my observations of modern methods of treatment had revealed that such cases are usually resistant to therapy.

### Techniques of acupuncture

For those of you who have not seen a demonstration of acupuncture treatments, let me give you a brief description of the technique. The needles are now usually made of stainless steel, are very thin and come in various lengths, from one to two inches long. They are inserted into the skin and muscles of the patient at specific points, known as meridian points, all over the body. There are one hundred and fifty to eight hundred points charted on the front and back of the body, the number varying from one school of acupuncture to another.

For the successful treatment of different diseases the acupuncturist must learn delicacy of execution, such as the depth and direction of placement of the needles; subtlety of manipulation and stimulation of the meridian points; and the proper combinations of meridian points on the body for various diseases.

Recent research has introduced electro-acupuncture, which seems to be much more efficient than the older method of manual stimulation of meridian points. The instrument used is a transistorised device powered by a nine-volt battery. Wires from this instrument are attached to the needles; again, according to the proper rules.

## *The status of acupuncture in Europe and the United States*

On my annual vacations to various parts of the world, I usually try to investigate acupuncture and consult with physicians who are practising it. Acupuncture was introduced into Europe as early as the seventeenth century, and practically every European country has an acupuncture society made up of doctors of medicine who use this therapy as an adjunctive treatment. About two thousand physicians practise it in France, and the French National Health Service acknowledges acupuncture and pays for the service.

However, I predict that unless the medical establishment and the public are better informed about acupuncture, including its limitations, this new therapeutic tool will very soon fall into disrepute and will be discredited and condemned.

Unscrupulous groups are setting up acupuncture clinics and institutes and are hiring so-called Asian acupuncturists, who have not had the proper background in medicine and surgery, to teach them where to insert the needles so they can claim to cure all diseases. In some cases, these places of deception and delusion are run like assembly lines, and hundreds of patients are seen daily. This cannot possibly be considered proper health-care management, and some states are now beginning to legislate against such facilities.

Hundreds of physicians in America are also being exploited by 'academies of acupuncture', or whatever euphemistic names they use. In various cities throughout the country, these promoters give three-day lectures and workshops in acupuncture, charging exorbitant prices to attend. There is absolutely no way that the techniques of acupuncture can be learned in three days – or even in three months.

This misuse of acupuncture must be stopped, or the yawning cultural gap between China and the West, which has been partially bridged by the Western interest in acupuncture, may be destroyed.

I want to remind the reader that acupuncture, with all its fascination, mystery and merits, is but one tool of treatment. Like the use of aspirin, indomethacin and other drugs, as well as physiotherapy and ultrasonics, it does not remove the cause of the disease. In my treatment for arthritis, nutrition is of primary importance; acupuncture and other modes of therapy are ancillary. I believe the following cases will show the effectiveness of this treatment.

NAME: Mr G. P.
AGE: 38
OCCUPATION: Pharmacist
RESIDENCE: Wyoming
DIAGNOSIS: Lumbar intervertebral disc syndrome
PREVIOUS MEDICATION: Aspirin, Darvon, codeine
FIRST VISIT: 2 November 1973
INTERVIEWED: 10 November 1973

'I had this back trouble since October 1968, with pains running down my right thigh. I took some pain medicine which helped me a little. But the condition progressed until it got so bad that I was sent to see some specialists in Salt Lake City.

'They took myelograms and told me that I had lumbar disc disease that was probably due to an old football injury.

My pains got worse, so they decided to operate on me. They removed a disc from the lumbar area in 1969. When I recovered from surgery, I felt good for about three months. One day I sat in a chair and I could not get up from it at all; I was in terrible pain. My doctor wanted to operate on me again in a region higher up on the back. But since the first operation didn't help me much, I felt the second operation would not either. I continued to take medicines to help the pain while I worked.'

[*When Mr G. P. came in to see me, recommended by another patient, he looked like an old man. He was almost unable to bend over and reported severe pains in his back and legs. I put him on the diet and gave him acupuncture treatments.*]

'One week later, I can get out of the chair, sit down and get up again. I can lift my leg and I can tie my shoes. These are things that I have not been able to do for three years. It sounds unreal, but it happened. It was very fortunate for me because no one knows what suffering is until they have had the kinds of pains that I have had.'

[*On Christmas 1973, Mr G. P. sent me a note and said, 'I am still doing very well. Hell of a diet to get used to. Merry Christmas.'*]

NAME: Mr A. C.
AGE: 51
OCCUPATION: Produce broker
RESIDENCE: Idaho
DIAGNOSIS: Osteoarthritis, cervical and thoracic spine; lumbar intervertebral disc syndrome
PREVIOUS MEDICATION: Aspirin, codeine, Darvon, Butazolidin, Percodan and others
FIRST VISIT: 15 March 1974
INTERVIEWED: 23 July 1974

'For about twenty years I have had pains in my neck and back. I have been to many doctors in Idaho. All the doctors told me that there was nothing that they could do about it. I took pain tablets day and night for years. Finally, one day I made up my mind to cut them all out. I learned to bear the pains and only took them if the pains were such that I could not stand it any more.

'In 1970 I had a car accident which flipped me over and crushed my right knee. I began having severe pains in the middle and lower parts of my back that I had never had before. I could not bend my knees at all, and could only bend from my waist. I was examined and treated at the University of Utah, but they too told me that there was nothing that could be done for me. I was then referred to the Mayo Clinic. Many X-rays and examinations were done there and the results were the same. Nothing could be done for me.'

[*On 15 March 1974, I started Mr A. C.'s treatment by putting him on the diet and giving him acupuncture treatments. At that time he weighed fourteen and a half stone. He now weighs thirteen stone.*]

'After the first three treatments I did not have any pains in my neck at all. After suffering twenty years with this pain this was great! My knee and back is not all well yet – but it doesn't hurt nearly like it did. It has been only six weeks since I started treatments.

'Before the car accident I was active in sports, even though I had the pains. I would play golf and take time off to ski. But since the accident in 1970, I was not able to participate in any sports at all. The other day, though, I played a whole game of golf. Of course, my score was not too good.'

NAME: Mr M. C.
AGE: 27
OCCUPATION: Unemployed
RESIDENCE: California
DIAGNOSIS: Sciatica, left side; osteoarthritis, left hip
PREVIOUS MEDICATION: Aspirin, codeine, Darvon, Percodan, Demerol, Dilaudid

FIRST VISIT: 5 April 1973
INTERVIEWED: 2 February 1974

'On 14 April 1967 I was run over by a bus. I was severely injured. I had a shattered pelvis with a dislocated head of the femur. I had agonising pains in my left hip from that moment on. I was confined in a hospital for one and a half months with a body cast and all kinds of contraptions on me. After my discharge from the hospital I must have consulted about twenty-five specialists – just trying to get rid of the constant and terrible pains. They started in my left hip, went down to the thigh and then to the leg. The doctors started me off with large doses of aspirin and codeine. I took so much of it that they had to give me antacids to counteract my stomach upset. About a year ago the pains were so bad that the doctors gave me all kinds of pain pills, Darvon, Percodan, Demerol and finally Dilaudid. I did not want to become an addict but the pains were so bad that I had to take the medicine.

'My mother heard about Dr Dong and made an appointment for me.'

[*Mr M. C. was a burly young man, six feet tall, with long hair, who limped into my office with the aid of a home-made cane. His attitude indicated frustration, disappointment and perhaps hostility. He had, no doubt, suffered much pain, agony and distress. If he was anti-establishment, he had a right to be. For here was a person who had been treated by many specialists for a period of six years with little result. He was a perfect example of the statement in* Medical Opinion: *'He's crippled by pain, hooked on medication, burdened by bills.'*

*After reading the medical history that he brought to my office I told Mr M. C. that there was no way in which I could possibly help him. At his insistence, because he claimed that I was his last hope, I explained my theory of treatment and the dietary regimen. I told him that if he expected to have any results, this programme that I was outlining to him would have to be adhered to minutely and religiously.*

*My previous experiences with this type of case have been unsuccessful for two reasons: first, multiple fractures, especially of the hip, and shortening of the leg, with intractable pains create abnormal conditions after healing that are very difficult to diagnose and treat. For six years after the accident Mr M. C. had been sent by the insurance company from one specialist to another for treatment, without result; and second, in the meantime, the patient had acquired a second disease, addiction to medication (Demerol and Dilaudid), which created another difficult medical problem not only physical, but also socio-psychological.*

*He agreed to follow my instructions and I started him on the diet and on acupuncture treatments.*]

'I weighed nineteen stone at the beginning of my treatments. Now I weigh twelve stone. After the first two treatments I had no pains or problems for three weeks – it was unbelievable. I don't know what happened, but I was able to sleep for eight hours a night and I could walk around flat-footed and move. Remember that my left leg is shorter due to the accident, and I could never walk flat-footed. I just had no problems. I had cut down on the pills a lot. Then, after three weeks, the pains came back again. I had to take the pills again, but after Dr Dong gave me another treatment, the pains disappeared like magic again. Each month, when I went in to see him, I improved. Today I have absolutely no pains. I have since moved to Chico, California, where I have taken a job. It is rather cold up there. I have been feeding the wood fire in my house with oak wood that I chop myself. You know how hard oak wood is. I have been working in the almond orchards chopping brush and I have been able to walk reasonable distances, like a mile or two. I have done more hard work in the last month than I have done in the last six years. And I take no pills at all.'

In this particular case, the Dong Diet and acupuncture and the cooperation of the patient produced a result that I never expected. This is the type of case that gives me immense joy and satisfaction.

# 9

# Summing up

Victor Hugo once said, 'There is nothing more powerful than an idea whose time has come.' In medicine the idea whose time has come is *nutrition's relation to diseases*. Medical scientists are at last beginning to realise that dietary prudence does play an important role in the aetiology and treatment of diseases. The public is beginning to be greatly concerned about nutrition. Patients are beginning to clamour for dietary instructions from their doctors. Consumers are beginning to pay attention to labels, and governments are studying food and nutrition in relation to public health.

Throughout this book I have quoted physicians and medical scientists who have definitively demonstrated that many diseases are nutritionally related. Heart disease, strokes, hypertension, diabetes, obesity and even cancer have been linked to improper diet. I have tried to explain my own profound concern about the relationship between nutrition and rheumatic diseases. I am confident that the medical community, especially those involved in the research and treatment of arthritis, will eventually stop ignoring this relationship.

### Nutritional research needed

It is important that we in the West no longer be nutritional illiterates. It is even more important that doctors and scientists remember that receptivity to new ideas and new avenues of research should be their fundamental consideration. I refer you again to those appalling statistics from U.S. government surveys showing that in 1966 there were seventeen million arthritics requiring medical care. The fact that this number increased by 1970 to twenty million two hundred and thirty thousand demonstrates that today's medical techniques for treatment and prevention of arthritis are abject failures.

These statistics alone should be enough to arouse serious scientific discourse and stimulate research as to whether or not there is validity in the hypothesis that dietary indiscretion may cause arthritis.

## Medicine is still an art – not an exact science

Earlier in this book I have described how, as a young doctor, I discovered a successful method of treating arthritis, but I was not ready to challenge medical orthodoxy because of my lack of experience. Now after all these years of experience, and with files of thousands of case histories of patients who have been successfully treated with my new therapy, I am still not challenging orthodoxy – or anyone's concepts. Experience in the medical world has given me humility. There are too many intangibles and unanswered questions in the practice of medicine. It is still an art – not an exact science.

My own experience with arthritis not only opened new horizons for me, but changed my entire perspective of life. I have received great satisfaction from the recovery of my many patients. Writing this book and recalling the various case histories has given me as much genuine pleasure as when these recoveries occurred.

## A new philosophy of life

When I was younger I wanted to shout from the housetops about my new great discovery on nutrition. However, maturity has given me a more philosophical point of view. I realise that I did not discover food and nutrition. Other doctors in the past have advocated common sense in eating.

When I was afflicted with arthritis, destiny had already prepared me for the position on its treatment that I would eventually take. As a boy I worked on a farm, harvesting crops of vegetables and fruit. I was a professional cook during many of my school vacations. I investigated the preparation of food in slaughter houses and canneries. Thus I was well prepared for putting into practice my new concept of the relationship of food to arthritis.

If my colleagues ignore nutrition in the treatment of their patients, there are extenuating circumstances. Medical school curricula do not include nutrition in their course of study. Our years of pragmatic training were, of course, necessary to learn the fundamentals of the human body and its pathology. But we also acquire a 'professorial syndrome' and become conformists. Although conformity is both confining and abrasive, most of us would not think of questioning the concepts of medical orthodoxy in the treatment of diseases – especially arthritis.

If and when the subject of nutrition is included in the medical curricula, merely giving lectures and teaching the theory of nutrition will be insufficient. In this respect, medicine is only a descriptive science. The students who become doctors will have much difficulty in translating this theoretical knowledge into practical advice for their patients. The theory of nutrition does not teach them how to cook or prepare a meal.

### Teaching nutrition to medical students is imperative

One of the most cherished experiences of my life was living at Taliesin West, the home of Frank Lloyd Wright, for two weeks. In 1954, I commissioned Mr Wright to design a building for me on Telegraph Hill in San Francisco. During that short stay in Arizona, I learned how the architectural genius trained his students.

His students are given a liberal education. Everyone is required to cultivate the land, plant and harvest crops, prepare and cook the food, serve other students and be served. In the evenings there were lectures in art, philosophy and literature, and on other occasions classical dancing and concerts were offered.

After the student was thoroughly inculcated with the humanities and the social and physical sciences, then, and only then, was he taught the fundamentals of architecture. Such an architect cannot help but be a superior one, well educated, cultured and conscientious.

We need a similar programme in medicine to give more practical experience to the student, especially in the fields of diet and nutrition. I wish all medical students were required during their summer vacations to learn agriculture, and to learn all about cooking and food preparation. In this way we could produce doctors who are superior in every phase of life. To paraphrase Dr Alfred D. Klinger, such doctors would then understand that nutrition is the cornerstone of life. They would know how to apply it properly to sustain the body and the mind. They would be able to teach their patients that the neglect of proper nutrition can cripple them.

In conclusion, I hope that the goals of this book have been accomplished. It was designed for the millions who are suffering from arthritis, but anyone can derive benefit from its information on diet and nutrition and how it is important to change the eating habits of people in the West to a more sensible pattern.

Remember also that this book and its dietary regimen is an auxiliary treatment for arthritis. You may have other physical conditions besides arthritis that require remedial measures, so you will still need the advice and care of your own doctor.

I hope that this book will be of value also to the doctors themselves, and even more importantly, that the understanding of the science of nutrition may improve the doctors' own health, so that they may continue to help others.

Mrs Banks and I have collaborated in translating my hypothesis of treatment into something definitive and comprehensive. In the section that follows, there are menus to make it easier to maintain the diet for longer periods of time, shopping and cooking tips to facilitate daily meal preparation, and many new recipes which will show you the wide variety of dishes you can prepare from the foods that are allowed on the Dong Diet.

# *The Mechanics*

# 10

# It's what you don't eat that counts

Before going into the how-to – the implementation – of the diet, let's clear up any misunderstanding of the basic principles. Some may think that simply consuming masses of fish and vegetables is going to do the trick – never mind the dab of hollandaise on the broccoli, never mind the little glass of orange juice without which it is impossible to start the day!

Let me say here and now, as firmly as possible: it isn't what you eat that does it as much as what you do *not* eat. Success depends on a strict adherence to the following lists, to the avoidance of the foods and additives designated as forbidden. The smallest infractions *do* make a difference, and there's no excuse for cheating. Dr Dong's diet is essentially an extremely simple one, and there's no reason in the world why it can't be a pleasant and satisfying one. Here is your list of do's and don'ts:

DO EAT:
  All seafood
  All vegetables, including avocados but excluding tomatoes
  Vegetable oils, particularly safflower oil
  Margarine (if possible, free of milk solids)
  Egg whites
  Honey
  Nuts, sunflower seeds, soybean products
  Rice of all kinds (brown, white or wild)
  Bread to which nothing on the 'Don't' list has been added
  Tea and coffee
  Plain soda water

Parsley, onions, garlic, bay leaf, salt
Flour (preferably the more nutritious unbleached and whole-grain)
Sugar (as little as your sweet tooth demands)
Chicken broth

## PERHAPS OCCASIONALLY:

Breast of chicken
A *small* amount of wine in cooking
A *small* drink of whisky or vodka
A small pinch of spicy seasoning such as curry powder
Noodles or spaghetti (since the amount of egg is relatively small and somewhat broken down in the cooking)

## DO NOT EAT:

Meat in any form, including broth
Fruit of any kind
Dairy products, including milk, cheese, and yogurt
Egg yolks
Vinegar, or any other acid
Pepper (most definitely) of any variety
Hot spices
Chocolate
Dry roasted nuts
Alcoholic beverages, particularly wine
Soft drinks (I've never found one without additives)
All additives, preservatives, chemicals, most especially monosodium glutamate. (One exception to this rule is lecithin in margarine.)

## EXCEPTIONS:

In addition to the very occasional exceptions allowed above, there are other unavoidable exceptions. Sensitivity to certain foods will vary from person to person; this must be determined by the individual. Allergies to certain seafoods, for instance, or accompanying diseases such as gout or colitis, will require a personal selection. In gout, or gouty arthritis, vegetables such as asparagus, spinach, artichokes, peas, beans, and mushrooms are possible offenders; in some colitis cases it might be necessary to cook all vegetables. In other words, take a common sense approach to what is essentially a common sense diet. For those allergic to shellfish I suggest a menu of fish and, later on, chicken or turkey breast. For those allergic to *all* seafood I can only suggest the white meat of chicken or turkey. These unfortunates must settle for deriving what benefit they can from a restricted regime. Again, it's not what you *do* eat that counts, it's what you *don't*.

At the outset the diet may seem formidable, I admit, for in the beginning even chicken breasts must be eliminated by those seriously affected by arthritis until there has been a definite improvement in their condition.

*The Arthritic's Cookbook* was written to introduce this diet to arthritis sufferers and to demonstrate how one could follow it and still have varied, tasty and even gourmet meals. In answer to many requests, in the pages that follow I am going to go into much more detail on various aspects of implementing the diet as well as share with you many additional recipes that I think are easy, economical and make marvellously satisfying dishes. For those new to the diet, I'm also going to give suggested menus to take you through the first week, followed by a plan to complete a month. Use your good common sense and experiment to determine what suits you best. Remember, we are all a little different, one from the other. Don't fight your individual tastes. The range of foods is wide enough to include *something* you like, I feel sure. There's no reason to force yourself to eat things you dislike. I'm not mad for beetroots, for instance. Bean sprouts, on the other hand, are a good food, economical and easy to grow in the kitchen window.

The suggested foods make up a sensible diet containing protein, vitamins, minerals and carbohydrates in digestible, acceptable form. The reduction in calories alone will be of immeasurable benefit; the fact that the body is being given only what it needs cannot help but improve the general health.

Obviously, however, not everyone will be able to adhere

to such a strict regime all the time, day in and day out. Some
office workers can take a packed lunch for instance; others
cannot. If a restaurant has no fish, try to get a sandwich
made of the white meat of chicken, and failing that, try for
tuna or peanut butter; it's often possible to get raw carrots
or celery to accompany the sandwich. Salads are a good
compromise; a tuna salad with a little mayonnaise, even if
it's not safflower-oil mayonnaise, is certainly going to be
preferable to a hamburger! You might settle for a vegetable
plate, as you can always make up the protein at the next
meal. Incidentally, remember that the white of the hard-
boiled egg is protein.

Experience will teach you what is most harmful to you
when you find you *must* deviate. I don't eat anything but the
salad and French bread on the airlines, as they use additives
to preserve the flavour of the rewarmed food. (You can
always have a nice little sandwich tucked away in your
carry-on bag, however.) I often find it very hard to explain
to a hostess who's gone to no end of trouble that I 'don't eat
meat' or 'can't have chocolate mousse', but which is more
important, an embarrassed apology or your lifelong health?

'Lifelong' is the keyword, of course. We all know we'll die
some-day; on the other hand, I'm sure there are very few
among us who don't like to feel we are doing all in our
power to maintain a long and healthy life span. As well as
eating the right food, you must eat the right amount of food.
We should give our bodies the necessary quantity of fuel,
no more, no less.

Above all, we must not gain weight. Think of a one-ton
car and imagine that after ten years' use it weighs a ton and a
half. Would you take this car out of the garage, expecting it
to stand up under the added strain? Our nutrition should be
looked upon in the same way; we should, as we age, consume foods that do not overload the body. Is it not preferable, perhaps essential, to allow the poor machine to function
unhampered?

The analogy between a car and our bodies is quite appropriate; many of the additives and detergents we are urged to
run through our car engines seem to result in a repair bill.

Just like a car, the body that's functioning well due to proper care will not deteriorate so fast – in other words, will live longer.

We should also remember that exercise is vital to the life process; exercise stimulates the circulation, helps throw off poisons through breathing and perspiration.

According to Dr Alex Comfort the human life span can be expanded by twenty to forty years and the chances of heart disease and cancer lessened. 'Longer life span is probably available now – for the young, if not the successful middle-aged, though they would gain.' He feels the way to do it is by simply limiting the calorie intake to sixty per cent of what we now eat. Or, he suggests, full-feeding for two days and fasting for one would accomplish the same thing. 'The foods to cut down are starch, sugar, dairy products and meat,' Dr Comfort points out. 'This applies to children as well as adults.' It is interesting to note that these are the very same items that are either eliminated or soft-pedalled in Dr Dong's diet for arthritics.

When you change to the diet, there's no need to feel that you must change your entire way of life. Growth and fulfilment need not stop just because of arthritis. Nor must the pleasures of life be set aside. Go out, get involved, broaden your horizons all around. Above all, live! Your arthritis will benefit, your world will look brighter, and you'll look brighter to all those around you.

# 11

# Planning and buying

After considerable enquiry and research, I've satisfied myself that it's quite possible to follow Dr Dong's regime anywhere you go. Easier, granted, where fresh fish and vegetables abound, but certainly not impossible in other places.

My food bills are most certainly below those of my meat-, fruit- and dairy-product-consuming friends. There's no doubt that in these days of soaring prices the food pound will stretch farther when expended for the less expensive fish – fresh *or* frozen – and vegetables – such as carrots, onions, potatoes, green beans and spinach. And the price of sugar hardly concerns us, as there is practically no use for it in this diet. Once you start using all your left-overs in soups, saving old bread for crumbs, even making your own bread if possible, I think you'll find you're way ahead financially as well as nutritionally.

The crowded, well-stocked refrigerator is no longer to be desired. The fresher your foods and the quicker they get to your table, the fewer chemicals you're likely to consume. And at today's prices, who can afford to throw away any spoiled food? On the other hand, it's good economics to plan, buy and cook ahead. If you have a busy week ahead or know you will be late getting home some night, it's a comforting feeling to know there's a fish casserole in the freezer waiting to be popped in the oven.

Allot a free morning to plan and cook ahead. Plot out your menus, assemble all your ingredients and cook everything more or less at once. Your bread or muffins can be rising while you peel the vegetables. You'll have to concentrate on watching a lot of things at once, and you'll feel somewhat like the chef of a famous restaurant overseeing his domain. Make your Chicken Broth, your Court Bouillon, and your Fish Stock (see the recipe section, pages 171–172), and store them either in the refrigerator or in the freezer, according to when you plan to use them. (They all freeze nicely.)

When buying vegetables, try to keep in mind that you should have some of the root vegetables, some of the leafy green, some raw and some cooked every day. It's usually possible, anywhere and at any time of year, to buy fresh carrots, celery, onions and potatoes. These can be kept on hand or cooked for use later, along with such vegetables as beetroots, green beans, brussels sprouts and courgettes. It's handy to have a ready supply of cold vegetables, slightly undercooked, to serve cold with an oil dressing either as a lunch dish or as a salad at dinner. I buy parsley in a sizable amount, chop it and keep it in a jar in the refrigerator. Parsley is rich in vitamins and minerals. It is also easy to grow either outdoors or in a pot in the kitchen window.

I prefer to steam vegetables, in order to save as many of the minerals and vitamins as possible. The water left in the bottom of the steamer is always saved for soup, as are all left-over vegetables, including celery and beetroot tops. Incidentally, cooking vegetables destroys the enzymes; this is why raw vegetables are especially valuable, and you will want to make use of both kinds.

This way of preparing food is really a return to the old basics and a simpler way of life, certainly more in keeping with the times than packaged foods and frozen dinners. But on top of that, when well prepared, this food has a simple elegance that's hard to beat.

The purchasing of these foods is of the utmost importance, of course, but before you do any buying, make a complete and careful check of all the labels already on your shelves for anything with additives or preservatives in it, and get rid of it.

Although the experts continually investigate the thousands of additives being used in food processing today, it is practically impossible to prove that an additive is safe for everyone.

And try as they may, no one can completely control food manufacture; the majority of food and drug inspectors are overworked, grossly underpaid public servants. The American Food and Drug Administration estimates that food poisoning has increased in the United States more than one thousand per cent since 1951. National Health Surveys report that digestive disturbances affect an estimated eight million people a year. To these figures, add the uncounted illnesses, allergies and health damage caused by additives, and you have a truly frightening picture.

We should be highly suspicious of any synthetic chemical that accumulates in the body. Although we don't yet know which chemicals cause or affect arthritis, we do know that it is a biochemical disturbance more than one of wear and tear. For this reason additional chemicals can only make the disease worse; what the well person may be resistant to can be extremely harmful to the sick person. In a previous chapter Dr Dong has listed some of the more commonly used additives, and it follows that we want to ingest as little of these as possible.

Geneticist James A. Crow wrote in an article entitled 'A Lethal Legacy', in *Science Year*, 1971:

It would be revealing to take a closer look at the incredible number of other man-made chemicals now found in our air, food, water and even our medicine cabinets. Some of these, such as drugs and food additives, we consume on purpose. Others like sulphur dioxide and nitrates, we take in helplessly in our polluted air and water. But we know little of how any of these chemicals affect us, because persons living today are the first to have ever been exposed to many of them. These chemicals threaten us in four ways: they can poison us, cause cancer, deform our unborn children in the womb and damage our hereditary material. . . .

In the past, we have been quite reckless in our ignorance. New chemicals have been widely used long before much was known about their long-term effects on either man or wildlife. In my view, many should have learned an important lesson from the cyclamate episode. Never again should we add a substance to the diet of an entire nation without first performing exhaustive tests to determine its potential for both short- and long-term harm to human beings.

Have we paid adequate attention to any of these warnings? How can the arthritic know just how much of his suffering has been chemically induced?

Environmentalist Colman McCarthy, in an article entitled 'Bon Chemical Appetit' in *The New Republic*, 30 November 1974, says:

Increased warnings are being sounded about the health dangers of many American foods. It's no longer just the carrot juice and yogurt groupies who worry, but others also, from school nutritionists to the nation's 104,000 dentists who must yank and fill the teeth rotted by 'fun foods'. It is not that science and chemicals are dirty words – such a dismissal ignores the many benefits to come from the labs – but that citizens have become an experimental control group.

Just when the public was beginning to realise that a lot of our food products were nutritionally worthless, the manufacturers started 'fortifying' them. The worthless food that already had artificial colour and flavour added now has vitamins added to persuade the consumer to buy. These vitamins, of course, do nothing to counteract the potential damage of the high levels of sugar, fat and salt. Dr Michael Jacobson, an MIT Ph.D. in microbiology, is with the Centre for Science in the Public Interest in Washington. Each year he appears at the annual meeting of American food technologists to award his Bon Vivant Vichyssoise Memorial Prize, a garbage can. In 1973 the winner was General Mills for Kaboom, Sir Gracefellow, Baron von Redberry and Franken Berry, all cereals containing thirty to fifty per cent sugar. The 1974 award went to Gerber's baby food. *The Wall Street Journal* of 13 January 1975, relates that the H. J. Heinz Co. is recalling about 600,000 boxes of instant dry baby cereal as a result of a *fourth* consumer complaint over metal particles found in the food.

We've gone into detail on these additives and preservatives to help you ascertain which foodstuffs are safe to buy and which aren't. You need to know which are more harmful than others. If you familiarise yourself with their names and initials, and then test your knowledge on the contents of your larder, you'll have an easier time. Your first few shopping trips are apt to be time-consuming, but you'll soon know what items to stay away from and what you can safely buy. Don't forget to take your glasses to the store! You must be able to see *everything* that's printed on the label!

Let's start with the basic items that one keeps on hand, such as bread, oil and margarine. Shopping for these things is easier today because, thanks to the increased interest in natural foods that began a few years ago, most major cities have health-food stores and many supermarkets now have sections devoted to such foods.

Starting with the good old staff of life, you'll want to look for breads that contain no dairy product or harmful preservative. In Britain there is no obligation to list the ingredients in bread, so you will have to do some research, find a baker or brand you can trust and stick to him or it. Some breads are actually offered as 'milk loaves' or 'milk enriched', and those of course you must avoid at all costs. Both branded wrapped loaves and the loose loaves you can buy at your local baker may contain additives, either added by the baker or mixed with the flour by the miller. For instance, citric acid is a permitted additive. Unpolluted breads are to be found in health-food stores, and nowadays increasingly in certain grocers and small bakers, but of course you are less likely to find them if you live outside a large city. *But* – and this is important – if the demand is great enough, the product will become available. If you and all your friends start bombarding the stores with requests for healthy breads, eventually you'll get them!

In the meantime, if you live in one of the areas where it's absolutely impossible to procure 'real' bread, I strongly suggest making it yourself. It really isn't all that complicated; it's mainly a matter of being around for the rising and kneading processes. In addition, and certainly to be considered in these times, you can make at *least* three loaves for the price of one shop-bought loaf. French bread, or a reasonable facsimile thereof, is very easy to make. I bake Wholewheat Bread (page 176) and Bran Muffins (page 175) about every two weeks and freeze what I don't need for immediate use.

After bread, the next staple items you'll want to look for are the oils and margarines. The use of oil is to be preferred over margarine. This does not mean margarine should be eliminated; it is simply used in moderation. The reason is that we try to stay with the foods that are highest in polyunsaturated fat, a type that is effective in reducing the cholesterol level in the blood. The hydrogenisation process that the oils must go through in the preparation of margarine considerably reduces the polyunsaturates. So try to condition yourself to use oil as much as possible, both in cooking and on your vegetables at serving time instead of margarine.

Safflower oil is highest in polyunsaturates and therefore preferable. Sunflower, soybean, corn, cottonseed, sesame and peanut oils come next. Corn oil is probably the most available and certainly quite acceptable if safflower oil cannot be found. On the other hand coconut oil, though used in many products and designated a vegetable oil, is actually more highly saturated than lard. Unfortunately, safflower oil is hard to find but, if your grocer doesn't have it, your chemist may. And it is carried in health-food stores. Like most other products, it will probably be much more expensive in chemists and health-food stores than in the supermarkets. Also, beware: oxidants such as BHT, BHA or propyl gallate may have been added to some brands, so read the label carefully before buying.

Safflower margarine will also be highest in the polyunsaturates, and therefore preferable. Again, you may not be able to find it and will have to settle for one of the corn oil margarines. You *are* likely to have trouble finding margarine without milk solids, but don't worry, because the amount used is not too great. It's much more important to remember to be moderate in the use of margarine. Combine it with oil whenever possible – when using it for browning in cooking, for instance.

Mayonnaise is a very useful adjunct to the diet. I find it useful in cooking as well as a necessity for salads. Dr Dong allows safflower-oil mayonnaise in spite of the fact that egg is among the ingredients. Here again, the amount is so negligible it may be ignored.

Peanut butter is a basic of the diet for me; but of course, this is a matter of individual taste.

You will need a supply of fish stock, and this you will have to make yourself (see recipe). Proprietary chicken broth, an absolute essential for a good deal of my cooking, is almost impossible to get without MSG; I have never found a tinned, packet or cube soup yet that didn't have additives. Again you will have to make your own, and I'll go more into your home-made supplies later.

Incidentally, it's worth remembering to check your supermarket for specials; there's always the chance of a good buy, particularly in some of the more expensive items.

When it comes to buying vegetables you'll of course want to buy the fresh produce available in season. I'm sure we're all aware by now of the importance of washing fresh produce well to remove any chemicals used to control pests, fertilisers, etc. When the vegetables you want are out of season, you can use a good frozen brand. Read the labels and eliminate all those that have anything added. Unfortunately, most 'convenience foods' are out. All those seductive ads on television that tell you how healthy this or that product is will have a list of chemicals on the label long enough, perhaps, to kill a horse! In certain instances I use a frozen vegetable even though I could use the fresh. I keep a supply of frozen chopped spinach on hand, for instance, for use in many recipes. It's so convenient that I forget how much better it would be if I used the fresh. The tiny frozen green peas are great in salad; I just put them in a sieve, pour boiling water over them and that's all the cooking they need.

We come now to buying fish and chicken. The latter is

easy, fresh is best, of course, but frozen will certainly do. If you can, try to buy chicken that hasn't been fed hormones or other undesirable things. You'll have to ask about the inclusion of hormones, however, as the law does not as yet require their listing on labels.

Fish is the backbone of this diet. It's our main source of quality protein, so if you don't like fish, just remember that fish likes *you*. Let me enumerate some of its nutritional properties: fish has a low-calorie, high-protein content; fishery products are the only sources of animal protein food in which the polyunsaturated fats are found in abundance; the protein of fish contains all of the biologically essential amino acids and is easily broken down by the digestive processes and readily available to the body. Fish contains many dietetically valuable minerals; iron, phosphorus, calcium, iodine, cobalt, copper, magnesium, potassium and other trace minerals necessary for the proper operation of the body. Fish is low in sodium content. Fish is rich in vitamins, particularly the B-complex series, which includes niacin, pantothenic acid, $B_{12}$, riboflavin, thiamine and pyridoxine. Convinced?

Obviously, if you have a fishmonger near you you'll be using it, and, equally obviously, with fresh fish available it will be easier to follow the regime. Ask the fishmonger to guide you in the selection and kinds and cuts of fish. Really fresh fish is firm to the touch, has shiny scales and bright eyes; it should smell strongly of the sea, never strongly fishy. Your choice will depend on whether you want to bake a whole fish, to grill fish steaks, to fry or poach. The main difference in kinds of fish is their fat content; salmon, trout and mackerel are higher in fat than sole, halibut and haddock. All shellfish are considered lean.

Availability and price are seasonal, of course.

Unfortunately, nowadays not everyone has an accessible fishmonger. However, nearly all supermarkets and grocers sell fish. Certain rules as to the handling and storing of frozen fish do prevail. Once thawed, fish must be used immediately, and should not be refrozen. Maximum storage life can be obtained by maintaining the temperature at zero degrees (Fahrenheit) or below and by providing adequate moisture-proof wrapping. If fish are placed directly in refrigerated space without protective treatment, a gradual loss of moisture will occur until the fish are shrunken and dried. Dehydration not only causes an unsightly appearance and alteration in texture but also results in loss of weight and flavour.

When you find yourself depending on frozen fish, you must find the brands that have been packaged with no additives and avoid all that have been precooked, breaded, or treated in any way. Among the packaged frozen fish are cod, sole, turbot, plaice, trout and haddock, as well as shellfish such as lobster, crab and shrimp. Of course, if you have a deep-freeze, you can freeze the fresh fish of your choice, and know that it's pure.

The best method of thawing fish is in your refrigerator, and as noted, it must be used immediately when thawed. The quickest way to thaw, but less desirable than the refrigerator method, is under cold running water, and the least desirable way is thawing at room temperature. This is because the thinner parts of the fish, such as the section near the tail, will thaw faster than other parts and may spoil if the thawing period is long.

Both fresh and frozen fish are sold in various forms, the cut more or less depending on the original size. Small fish are usually sold whole or drawn; medium fish whole or drawn and with the head, tail and fins removed; and larger fish are sold filleted or as steaks. The advantage of the fillet, of course, is that there are practically no bones. Frozen fish are usually filleted.

Servings of fresh and frozen fish generally are based on portions of one-third to one-half pound for each person. Of course when estimating amounts you must take into account the edible portions of whatever form you're considering.

# 12

## And the cooking . . .

Fish cookery, both of the fresh and the frozen, has some very definite maxims. Fish must always be cooked gently. Low heat is best, and overcooking is absolutely fatal to the delicate flavour and texture. You really must attend to business when you're cooking fish; you must be on hand to end the cooking at the very instant of completion. Another good rule to remember is that fish cooking is *moist* cooking. You are always cooking it either in a broth such as a Court Bouillon (page 171), baking it covered to retain the juices, basting it, or sautéeing it very quickly.

So, fish can be grilled, poached, fried, sautéed or baked. Small fish such as trout are best dredged in flour and fried in safflower oil. Mackerel, salmon, sole, turbot and the like can be poached whole or filleted, a method I find highly satisfactory. I think very few things can equal a piece of poached turbot with a pat of margarine melting on it.

A good, simple way of cooking frozen fish is by poaching. Haddock can, after poaching, be cut into pieces and made into a casserole. Cover with a cream sauce made by sautéeing chopped onions in oil, working in a little flour and margarine, cooking slightly, and then thinning with a bit of the poaching water. Bake with some breadcrumbs sprinkled on top and perhaps seasoned with a herb such as tarragon or basil. This dish can be a very good, inexpensive standby.

Another easily prepared fish if you can find it is rock turbot. It has no scales, and the skin will slide off very much like that of the eel. And it can be prepared in chunks because the meat falls away from the bones very easily. However,

you may prefer it in steaks or fillets. Either way, dry the
pieces well, dip them in egg white slightly beaten with a little
water, and cornstarch or flour, then fry them in your oil-
and-margarine mixture. You can add chopped parsley to the
browned oil to pour over the fish, or you might like a
mixture of chopped fresh herbs. For a whole fish, try Rock
Turbot with Herbs (page 191) or Rock Turbot Martigues
(page 192).

Steaks of any of the larger fish such as haddock can be
grilled, and all the larger fish can also be baked in a variety
of ways. The shellfish are all delicate and should be handled
accordingly. They can be either simmered a few minutes or
sautéed just till they turn colour.

Don't destroy the marvellous flavour and texture of fish
with a lot of herbs and seasonings; just the lightest touch is
needed, only enough to bring out the natural flavours.
Incidentally, one need hardly salt fish at all, for fish are rich
in natural salts. Fish lends itself to good cooking better than
anything else I can think of, and perhaps this is why the
French make so much use of their *fruits de mer*!

Obviously, frozen fish is never going to be as good as fresh
when simply grilled, but I've found that frozen sole, halibut,
haddock and trout are all good when handled properly to
disguise the change in texture. Frozen fish is apt to be dry
due to the loss of moisture, and so must be prepared in a
way that will replace that moisture.

The main point to remember is to defrost the fish slowly
and thoroughly. Remove it from the package, place it on a
plate, and let it defrost slowly in the refrigerator. When it's
completely unfrozen and you can separate the pieces without
breaking them, lay the fish on paper towels and pat it
thoroughly dry. It's then ready to prepare in much the same
way as you would with fresh. As I said, I have good luck
poaching it, particularly sole, and serving it either with a
sauce or flaking it into a casserole with a cream sauce.
Amandine – sautéeing it in browned oil and margarine with
almonds – is another good way.

Fish cookery is a Mediterranean speciality, particularly in
Provence, and some of their methods for handling their

dryish fish lend themselves nicely to preparing frozen fish. For instance, in Provence a whole fish is placed in a dish, covered with their marvellous olive oil, and allowed to stand in the sun for several hours. It's then removed from the oil and grilled. Halibut steaks and the other large varieties of frozen fish can be improved by an oil marinade. I season my safflower oil with a little good olive oil, perhaps adding a herb or two such as fennel or thyme, and let the defrosted fish rest in it for an hour or so – not necessarily in the sun, however! I also find that just brushing the oil on the fillets before grilling helps counteract the dryness.

As a general rule you can cook frozen fish in any of the ways you'd prepare it fresh, but some methods are just better for preserving the flavour and texture. There are many recipes in *The Arthritic's Cookbook* for cooking frozen sole that could be adapted to other frozen fish fillets. But do be careful to thaw your frozen fish carefully, dry it as suggested, and above all, be extra careful not to overcook.

At the risk of sounding like a nut on the subject of over-cooking, I'm going to extend that maxim to frozen vegetables as well. I prefer all vegetables slightly undercooked, both to preserve their flavour and texture and to preserve as many vitamins and minerals as possible. Potatoes, of course, are an exception. Is there anything worse than an underdone baked potato?

If only a single member of the family is on Dr Dong's diet, that naturally presents difficulties for the cook. We all know what a nuisance it is to prepare a special menu for one person. The cook gets tired of it, and someone usually gets short shrift. But isn't it possible to explain to the other members of the family the enormous benefits to be derived from this healthy, balanced diet? The man in the family especially will profit. A woman I know, an arthritic, decided simply to start cooking this way for herself and her husband without mentioning it to him. After he'd been thriving on it for some time, he told her he'd heard about 'this fish-and-vegetable diet for arthritis' and suggested she try it. 'My dear,' she said, 'I've been on it for three months, and so have you!' After he'd recovered from his surprise, he realised that he felt better than he'd felt in years, his weight was down, and he'd *enjoyed* it!

However, if such cooperation is impossible, it is not diffi-cult for the arthritis sufferer to have his portion of fish or chicken cooked his way, to have the vegetables that would be served in any case, and to skip any dairy products and fruits. But do try to protect the rest of the family from harmful additives and preservatives. We just don't know enough about the evils of these modern poisons. Who knows what unknown troubles you may be saving them from in later life? Try, too, to provide a good balance of protein, minerals and carbohydrates, soft-pedaling the unnecessary, fattening items. Let raw carrots and celery gradually replace the Danish pastry and apple pie.

# 13

# But what do you eat for breakfast?

Breakfast means tea and toast to me, but I realize that for many it's the most important meal of the day. Some may need protein to support a physically active day; some may require a bit of sugar (I feel I do, so I have a bit of honey on my toast). It's quite possible to satisfy all tastes!

However, the first habit to break is that glass of orange juice. *Forget* about fruit and fruit juices; simply put them out of your mind. Try substituting a glass of carrot juice. It is a fine source of vitamins and easy to make in a blender. If you feel the day isn't off to a proper start without cereals, by all means have it, but you'll have to get used to eating it without milk or cream. Believe it or not, a little chicken broth isn't bad over cereal, or for cooked cereal, try a little melted margarine.

Here again I must warn you to read the labels. Only a few of the dry cereals are free of additives. Many cereals contain BHT, among them Wheaties, Kellogg's Corn Flakes and Rice Krispies. Quaker Oats and Shredded Wheat, however, have no additives. Incidentally, the ratio of carbohydrates to protein is high in all the cereals and should be borne in mind when weight is a factor.

For those of you accustomed to starting the day with an egg, a delicious Egg-White Omelette (page 174) should satisfy. Try it different ways till you find a variation that suits you – with chopped parsley, with a combination of herbs and chives, with thinly sliced celery or green pepper, or even with nuts. My favourite is a combination of thinly sliced spring onions and slivers of green pepper. Add a slice or two of wholewheat toast and you have a good, protein-rich breakfast. For those who feel the need for even more protein there's always kippers, haddock, or perhaps a piece of chicken or creamed tuna on toast.

Muffins are good for breakfast; home-made Bran Muffins are delicious, particularly with honey. Do a little experimenting. Treat yourself on Sunday morning to French toast and real honey syrup. Simply soak wholewheat bread in egg white, slightly beaten with a little water, until the bread soaks up the liquid. Brown the bread crisply in a frying pan, melt a small pat of margarine on top, add the honey and enjoy with lots of good coffee. Who can complain of this as an accompaniment to the Sunday paper?

# 14

# Now we start

By now you should be all primed with positive thinking and determination. Following this regimen is likely to mean a complete shift in life-style for most people. I have made up a thirty-day menu for those who want definite guidelines. If you meticulously follow this day after day for three meals a day, I don't think you'll have *time* to have arthritis, let alone anything else! You'll be too busy shopping for the ingredients and cooking. However, with some adjustments for leftovers, for availability, and for personal taste, you should then be able to follow the diet on your own. Remember, the white meat of chicken is allowed no more than once a week. And if you are an extreme sufferer, substitute fish for the breast of chicken for about a year. And remember, no deviations whatsoever at any time!

It's probably safe to assume that the great majority of people starting out on the diet are somewhat overweight and could stand to lose about ten pounds. With the elimination of carbohydrates, this can be done in the first two weeks. Just stay away from the bread and potatoes and rice for the first week, substitute carrots or celery, and concentrate on how great it will be not to have to worry about weight again. (And I mean never again. I'm willing to wager that if you stay on the diet six months you'll never go back to your old ways.) For those few people fortunate enough to be truly thin, French bread, muffins, and other things of this sort may be added during this first week.

Incidentally, unbleached flour and brown rice are generally thought to be superior nutritionally. I also feel it is preferable to have a low sugar intake. For this reason, you won't find many desserts in the menus, as I hope you'll lose your craving for sweets when your body is fed by a balanced combination of foods. Moderation has never been one of my favourite words, but it's vitally important when applied to nutrition. Don't use too *much* margarine, don't drink too *much* coffee, don't use too *many* herbs! And above all, use salt sparingly. Generally speaking, a reduction of salt is found to be helpful.

The following outline of a thirty-day plan is not intended to be followed meticulously and to the letter. It's quite likely it contains some foods you don't care for at all, and there may be some recipes too complicated for you to want to bother with. If there's something you particularly like, repeat it as often as you wish as a substitute for something else on the menu. For instance, for those who can't get fresh fish, the Tuna Casserole can be repeated. As to amounts, this must be left up to the discretion of the individual. A great strapping man who is going off to a hard day's work is obviously going to need more nourishment than a quiet elderly lady whose total game plan may be a walk around the block. Again, the magic word is moderation!

# 15

# The one-month menu plan

## FIRST WEEK

### First Day

Breakfast: Egg-White Omelette,* one thin piece of French bread toast

Lunch: Fish salad ($\frac{1}{2}$ tin white fish [e.g. cod or haddock] with chopped celery, spring onion and safflower mayonnaise)

Dinner: Cup of hot fish stock generously sprinkled with chopped parsley
Fish Casserole I*
Green Beans

### Second Day

Breakfast: Two medium stalks of celery stuffed with a reasonable amount of peanut butter

Lunch: Spinach-Shrimp Salad*

Dinner: Scalloped Oysters*
Steamed carrots
Braised Courgettes
Small handful of walnuts (Walnuts are high in poly-unsaturates; other nuts are all right depending on allergies)

### Third Day

Breakfast: Kippers, a thin piece of French toast

Lunch: Large bowl of vegetable soup (chopped vegetables cooked in chicken broth)

* Recipes to follow.

Dinner: Small green salad with oil, dill and salt dressing
    Sole Chinoise*
    Rice, with a dab of margarine
    ¼ head of cabbage, steamed, with a dab of margarine

*Fourth Day*

Breakfast: Egg-White Omelette* made with herbs, a thin
    piece of toast
Lunch: Vegetable Pancakes*
Dinner: Cup of chicken broth
    Brochette Provencal* (using frozen fish if necessary)
    Green beans with sage
    Tiny handful of almonds

*Fifth Day*

Breakfast: 1 slice of French Toast,* with 1 dessertspoon of
    honey
Lunch: Medium helping of Organic Salad*
Dinner: Sole Meunière*
    Ratatouille*
    Dr Dong's Basic Rice Pudding,* with brown sugar

*Sixth Day*

Breakfast: Egg-White Omelette* made with spring onions
    and parsley
Lunch: Gado Gado*
Dinner: Tuna Soufflé*
    Fresh steamed spinach
    Small baked potato, with a dab of margarine
    1 Almond Oatmeal Cookie*

*Seventh Day*

Breakfast: Chopped hard-boiled egg whites in a thin White
    Sauce* on a piece of thin toast
Lunch: Clam Chowder*
Dinner: Dr Dong's Chicken*
    Rice Pilaf with Vegetables*
    1 plain biscuit with peanut butter

With the completion of the first week you should begin to feel somewhat adjusted to the regime. Your appetite should be satisfied; your general feeling should be one of well-being, although it's too soon to expect relief from the pains of arthritis. Since Dr Dong feels that thirty days is a reasonable test, you must not feel discouraged if there's no relief sooner. However, if at the end of a month's time there's no relief *whatsoever*, it's probable that your problem has other facets. The plan is, as I said, adjustable. If there are foods not to your liking, substitute another from the plan; if one doesn't agree with you for one reason or another, try another. Portions should be moderate, and always use a minimum of margarine. And keep checking your weight.


## SECOND WEEK

*First Day*

Breakfast: Dr Dong's Basic Rice Pudding*
Lunch: Fish Aspic Salad,* with a few carrot sticks
Dinner: Corn Soup*
  Tuna Surprise*
  Sautéed Aubergine

*Second Day*

Breakfast: Whole-grain cereal, melted margarine and brown
    sugar
Lunch: Celery Victor,* sprinkled with hard-boiled egg white
Dinner: Small green salad with oil, dill weed, and garlic salt
    dressing
  Chicken Pie*
  Small serving of Angel Cream*

*Third Day*

Breakfast: Muffin, margarine, and honey
Lunch: Cooked vegetable salad
Dinner: Salmon steak
  Brussels sprouts, small white pickling onions
  Rice
  A few walnuts

*Fourth Day*

Breakfast: Egg-White Omelette* made with slivered green
    pepper, a thin piece of toast
Lunch: Peanut butter and fresh bean sprout sandwich
Dinner: Sole or Flounder Bonne Femme*
  Steamed carrots and peas
  Dr Dong's Basic Rice Pudding,* with brown sugar

*Fifth Day*

Breakfast: Creamed hard-boiled egg whites on thin toast
Lunch: Leek and potato soup
Dinner: Prawns sautéed in safflower oil and margarine
  Dollar Potatoes*
  Green Beans
  1 or 2 Sesame Seed Cookies*

*Sixth Day*

Breakfast: 1 Walnut Waffle,* with a dessertspoon of maple
    syrup
Lunch: Vegetables with Herbs*
Dinner: Chicken with Broccoli*
  A small handful of walnuts (or other)

*Seventh Day*

Breakfast: Kippers or sardines, a piece of toast
Lunch: Clam Salad*
Dinner: Half an avocado
  Fish Casserole II*
  Spinach, small white pickling onions in White Sauce*
  1 Almond Oatmeal Cookie*

## THIRD WEEK

*First Day*

Breakfast: Muffin, with honey
Lunch: Chinese Omelette*
Dinner: Salad with mixed greens and raw vegetables
  Shellfish Soup*
  French bread, margarine

*Second Day*

Breakfast: Tuna in thin White Sauce * on toast
Lunch: Salade Niçoise *
Dinner: Chicken in a Wok*
   Cold artichokes with safflower mayonnaise
   1 Sesame Seed Cookie *

*Third Day*

Breakfast: French Toast * with honey
Lunch: Fresh bean sprout and avocado sandwich
Dinner: Steamed mackerel with soy-garlic-ginger sauce
   Baked potato
   Green beans
   A handful of walnuts

*Fourth Day*

Breakfast: Pancakes, * with honey or syrup
Lunch: Shrimp salad with safflower mayonnaise
Dinner: Chicken Broth * with herbs and rice
   Tuna Pie *
   1 Almond Oatmeal Cookie *

*Fifth Day*

Breakfast: Porridge (made with water, not milk, and served
    with a little melted margarine and brown sugar)
Lunch: Chicken sandwich
Dinner: Artichoke
   Sole or Flounder sautéed in oil and margarine, with
    chopped parsley
   Rice
   Creamed Spinach *

*Sixth Day*

Breakfast: Egg-White Omelette * made with slivered celery
Lunch: Organic Salad *
Dinner: Bourride (Fish Stew) *
   Green salad

*Seventh Day*

Breakfast: Walnut Waffles with Syrup*
Lunch: Courgette Fritata*
Dinner: Cod with Mushrooms*
  Polenta*
  Broccoli


## FOURTH WEEK

*First Day*

Breakfast: Dorothy's Arabic Bread,* margarine, and honey
Lunch: Poached scallops or steamed clams
Dinner: Chicken Breasts Chinoise*
  Baked potato
  Creamed Cabbage*
  Small slice Mayonnaise Cake*

*Second Day*

Breakfast: Kippers, thin toast
Lunch: Crab and Rice Salad*
Dinner: Baked Haddock Steak*
  Rice with margarine and chopped parsley
  Fresh asparagus or green beans
  2 Marcaroons*

*Third Day*

Breakfast: Muffin with honey
Lunch: Fish Salad*
Dinner: Cold Cucumber Soup*
  Fish Creole*
  Rice
  Green beans
  A few nuts

*Fourth Day*

Breakfast: Egg-White Omelette* with slivered onions
Lunch: Chicken sandwich, carrot sticks

Dinner: Fish Soufflé
  Mixed green salad
  French bread
  Dr Dong's Basic Rice Pudding* with honey

*Fifth Day*

Breakfast: ¼ tin tuna in thin White Sauce* on toast
Lunch: Beetroot soup, a slice of French bread
Dinner: Baked Shrimp*
  Sautéed green peppers
  Baked carrots

*Sixth Day*

Breakfast: Muffin
Lunch: Cold vegetable plate: boiled potato, beets, carrots,
    and courgettes, marinated together
Dinner: Bourride (Fish Stew)*
  French bread
  Zabaglione*

*Seventh Day*

Breakfast: French Toast,* syrup or honey
Lunch: Chicken sandwich in Dorothy's Arabic Bread,* with
    safflower mayonnaise
Dinner: Clam broth
  Fish Casserole II*
  Baked potato
  Fresh spinach
  A few nuts

# 16

# For special occasions

There are special occasions in everyone's life. The fact that you're coping with your arthritis through diet need not preclude your celebrating these occasions. The following menus are simply suggestions to stimulate your imagination. I'm sure you can fill in with items from the thirty-day plan, or improve on these menus with some inventions of your own.

I prefer to entertain no more than six or eight at a time, so my ideas for dinner parties are mainly geared to groups of this size. Obviously, the recipes are expandable, however.

Don't tell your guests they're eating an arthritic's diet *before* dinner. Wait till they've complimented you on a delicious meal, and then break the good news to them that they've had a healthy, non-fattening, cholesterol-free dinner.

BUFFET SUPPER FOR EIGHT OR TEN

To pass with the cocktails you don't drink:

Bowls of peanuts, walnuts, almonds
Herbed Toast *
Aubergine Caviar *
Stuffed Vine-Leaves *

On a tray as a first course:

Pass cups of Carrot and Tarragon Soup *

For dinner, arrange on the buffet:

Turkey Breast with Tuna Sauce on Rice *
A plate of cold cooked vegetables marinated in oil, dill
and garlic salt: green beans, peas, beetroots, courgettes,
carrots, decorated with cocktail tomatoes and ripe
olives
Long hot loaf of French bread, sliced and margarined
Angel Food Cake *
Espresso coffee

## SMALL SEATED DINNER

With cocktails:

Shrimp Pâté * served with toast rounds

Dinner:

Chinese Eggdrop Soup *
Salmon en Croute *
Broccoli and baby carrots
French bread
Walnut Dessert *

## SUNDAY NIGHT SUPPER

I particularly like Sunday nights. It's a nice informal time
to entertain, and the food can be simple and undemanding
without sacrificing appeal. On Sunday nights in winter I
might serve Bouillabaisse * in big earthenware bowls, a huge
green salad, and lots of hot, crusty French bread. On a
Sunday night in summer, when my crop of fresh basil is
available (it's easy to grow in pots), I like to serve a big plate
of spaghetti a la vougole,* a green salad, crusty French
bread and Zabaglione * for dessert. And, of course, coffee.

* There's a recipe in *The Arthritic's Cookbook*.

## SUNDAY LUNCH

In Summer Sunday noon is a time we like to have people
out from the city to lunch out-of-doors. I keep it simple, and
serve things that can be prepared ahead.

  Cold Cucumber Soup*
  Chicken Breasts Mary Elizabeth*
  Green salad
  Macaroons* and coffee

## BIRTHDAY DINNER

  Fresh oysters
  Poached Salmon with Green Mayonnaise*
  Fresh asparagus
  Wild rice
  Angel Food Cake* and coffee

## LUNCHEON PARTY

  Poached Sole Chaudfroid*
  Spinach-Stuffed Mushroom Caps*
  Vanilla Soufflé*

An alternative main dish might be Avocado Stuffed with
Chicken Salad.*

# *Recipes*

# 17

# Basic needs

## CHICKEN BROTH

I make my chicken broth one of two ways: When I poach chicken breasts, which I do fairly often to use for chicken salad, sandwiches or serving with a sauce, I save the broth they were poached in. It is rich and usually flavoured with a little tarragon and perhaps a bay leaf and some salt. The other way I make it is by dropping a couple of chicken legs in a pot, covering them well with water, and simmering till I feel I've got all the chicken flavour I can out of the legs. Here again I usually add a few herbs – bay leaf, thyme, marjoram – depending upon what I'm using the broth for.

## COURT BOUILLON

This basic liquor for poaching fish can be made ahead of time. Chop a couple of carrots, a large celery stalk, and about two onions into three cups of water. Add a bay leaf, a good pinch of thyme and several sprigs of parsley. Sea salt is a good addition to the flavour of fish. Simmer the mixture for about thirty minutes and strain before using. The addition of a glass of white wine will improve this bouillon, but use it only after you really feel completely well.

## FISH STOCK

Ask the fishmonger for the bones and trimmings when your fish is prepared. Put them in three cups of water with a sliced onion, a handful of parsley, salt (or sea salt), and simmer for about thirty minutes. Strain. Here again wine is a nice addition, but only if your arthritis is no longer giving you pain.

## WHITE SAUCE

1 *dessertspoon margarine*
1 *dessertspoon flour*
¾ *cup chicken broth, fish stock, or water (depending on what you want to use the sauce with and what you have on hand).*

Blend the margarine and flour over low heat to make a roux. Let it bubble a few minutes, then gradually add the chicken broth, fish stock or water.

# Breakfasts, eggs and breads

## FRENCH TOAST

Take a thin slice of French or regular bread made without
eggs, butter or additives. Soak in a slightly beaten egg white
till it is absorbed, and brown in a small amount of safflower
oil. Serve with a thin pat of margarine and honey.

## PANCAKES

1 *cup flour*
1 *dessertspoon sugar*
1 *dessertspoon baking powder*
½ *teaspoon salt*
1 *egg white*
¾ *cup water*
1 *tablespoon safflower oil*

Sift the dry ingredients together; beat the egg white lightly
and add the other wet ingredients and mix thoroughly.
Combine the wet and dry ingredients and stir just enough to
mix together. The batter should be lumpy. Cook in a heavy
frying pan.

## WALNUT WAFFLES WITH SYRUP

1¼ *cups flour*
2 *teaspoons baking powder*
½ *teaspoon salt*

1¼ cups water
2½ tablespoons safflower oil
2 egg whites, stiffly beaten
½ cup chopped walnuts

Sift the dry ingredients together, add the water and oil, and mix thoroughly till smooth. Fold in the stiffly beaten egg whites and pour the batter into a waffle iron. (It's worth treating yourself to one for the extra variety it provides).

## CHINESE OMELETTE

1½ tablespoons chopped Chinese cabbage and/or bean sprouts
Safflower oil to cover bottom of pan
1 4½-oz tin shrimp, or equal amount fresh shrimp (or prawns)
5 egg whites
1 teaspoon cornstarch
Soy sauce
Pinch of sugar

Sauté the vegetables slowly in the oil until just crisply tender; add the shrimp. Meanwhile, break the egg whites into a bowl. Do not beat them! Gently stir the vegetables into the egg whites in the bowl. When the mixture is well stirred, drop by the ladleful into the oiled pan, making small omelettes about six inches across. Use a spatula to keep them from spreading; they will take form almost immediately. Cook them slowly till brown; turn and brown on the other side. Meanwhile put the cornstarch in a bowl with a little cold water; add some soy sauce and a pinch of sugar; mix well. After the omelettes are removed from the pan, pour this mixture into the pan and stir carefully till it becomes a clear, glazelike sauce to serve over the omelettes.

## EGG-WHITE OMELETTE

Heaped dessertspoon slivered spring onion, celery or green
    pepper, or combination thereof
1 dessertspoon safflower oil

2 *egg whites per person*
*Pinch salt*

Sauté the vegetable of your choice lightly in the oil, preferably using a Teflon pan. This will take a very short time.
Remove the vegetables from the oil with a slotted spoon,
stir into the egg whites, and add salt. Do not beat; just stir
around gently to mix. Slide the mixture into the still-hot
pan and sauté a very short time, just enough to brown lightly.
Turn, brown and serve. You can make this in any number of
variations; I'm very fond of onions and often make an
omelette with lots of sliced mild onions as a luncheon dish.

## BRAN MUFFINS

2 *oz yeast, dissolved in* 4 *tablespoons lukewarm water* (*be sure
   your yeast is fresh*)
$\frac{3}{4}$ *cup very warm water*
1 *teaspoon salt*
2 *teaspoons honey* (*optional – I prefer it without*)
1 *cup bran*
1$\frac{1}{2}$ *cups stone-ground wholewheat flour*
1$\frac{1}{2}$ *cups unbleached white flour*
2 *level tablespoons soft margarine*

Combine the dissolved yeast, water, salt, honey and bran in
a large bowl. Mix the flours together in a separate bowl, and
gradually beat half of the flour into the bran mixture. Cover
the bowl and allow to rise in a warm place for one and a half
hours. Beat in the margarine and add the rest of the flour,
reserving just under half a cup for the board. Turn out on to
the board and knead until smooth. Don't skimp on the
kneading! Pat the dough out, spreading till it's about three
quarters of an inch thick. Cut into three-inch rounds; cover
on the board for about an hour. Cook in a lightly oiled, hot
(but not too hot!) heavy frying pan for twelve or thirteen
minutes, turning once. To serve, split and toast.

## DOROTHY'S ARABIC BREAD

4 *heaped cups unbleached wheat flour*
4 *tablespoons stone-ground wholewheat flour*
½ *teaspoon salt*
1¾ *cups water*
1½ *oz dried yeast*
1½ *tablespoons safflower oil*

Sift together the flours and salt. Heat the water to 110 degrees (you'll have to guess if you haven't a thermometer). Pour some of the warm water into a large mixing bowl and add the yeast and the oil. Alternately add the flour and water, mix well and knead on a bread board for about ten minutes. Let rise in a warm place for an hour and a half, then roll out into a long roll, and slice into fourteen equal parts. Take each piece and roll it out three quarters of an inch thick. Place each piece on a four-inch square of foil, and let rise for another hour. Preheat the oven to 500 degrees (gas No. 9), brush each piece with oil, and bake for nine minutes on the lowest rack in the oven. (You can probably bake four at a time.)

## WHOLEWHEAT BREAD

2 *teaspoons salt*
1 *tablespoon margarine*
1½ *cups warm water*
2 *oz fresh yeast, dissolved in 4 tablespoons lukewarm water*
1¾ *cups unsifted all-purpose flour (unbleached)*
2¼ *cups unsifted stone-ground wholewheat flour*

Mix the salt and margarine with the water. Add the yeast and the all-purpose flour. Start adding the wholewheat flour slowly, and when all is mixed in, turn out on to a floured board. Knead until the dough is smooth and elastic, from five to ten minutes. Place in an oiled bowl, cover with a dish towel, and place in a pan of hot water in an unlighted oven for about one and a half hours. It should double in bulk.

Knead again, and let rise again in the same way. Shape into two loaves and place in two oiled 9 × 5-inch loaf pans. Let rise once again till double in size. Bake at 400 degrees (gas No. 5) for forty-five minutes. Let cool on a wire rack.

# Appetisers

## STUFFED VINE-LEAVES

2 *or 3 onions, finely chopped*
¾ *cup mixed white and wild rice*
8 *spring onions, chopped*
4 *tablespoons chopped parsley*
1 *tablespoon dill weed*
3 *tablespoons finely chopped walnuts*
8 *tablespoons olive oil mixed with eight tablespoons water*
*Vine-leaves*

Sauté the onions in a little olive oil, then mix together all the ingredients except the vine-leaves, and simmer for about ten minutes. Rinse the leaves carefully to remove the brine. Wrap each leaf around about a teaspoon of the rice mixture and put them in a large frying pan in one layer. Pour over them the olive oil and water mixture. Put a heavy lid over the rolls to keep them from unwrapping, and simmer for forty-five minutes.

## AUBERGINE CAVIAR

*A green pepper, seeded and chopped*
*An onion, chopped*
1½ *tablespoons olive oil*
*A clove garlic, crushed*
*A baked aubergine, peeled and seeded*
*Salt to taste*

Sauté the green pepper and onion in the olive oil; add the garlic and aubergine. Salt to taste, and serve with crisp, thin wedges of toasted French bread.

## HERBED TOAST

Chop equal parts of parsley, tarragon, and chives very fine. Mix with a quarter-pound of margarine and spread on very thin slices of French bread. Toast in a 350-degree oven (gas No. 4) till brown and crisp.

## SHRIMP PÂTÉ

Put a half pound of small cooked shrimp in the blender with eight tablespoons olive oil. Puree, then add another cup of oil, salt to taste and a dash of paprika. Cover and refrigerate. Serve on a plate with melba toast. This recipe makes quite a lot but you can easily adjust it for a smaller amount.

# Soups

## BOURRIDE (FISH STEW)

*an onion, chopped*
*1 tablespoon olive oil*
*2 leeks, chopped*
*3 carrots, sliced*
*a celery heart, chopped*
*¼ cup chopped parsley*
*3 potatoes, peeled and sliced*
*a pound of cod fillets (or whatever firm-fleshed fish is available)*
*1½ cups hot fish stock (see page 171)*
*a dessertspoon of white wine (optional)*
*Salt to taste*
*Slices of French bread*
*Cooking oil*
*Margarine*
*¾ cup mayonnaise mixed with 1 garlic clove, crushed.*

Sauté the chopped onion in the olive oil, add the rest of the
vegetables, and stir over low heat for five minutes. Place the
fish on top of the vegetables, cover tightly, and simmer over
very low heat for half an hour, or until the vegetables are
tender. Remove the fish to a warm dish, pour the vegetables
into a blender, and puree till smooth. Pour the puree into a
tureen, add the hot fish stock slowly, plus a dessertspoon of
white wine if you wish, and salt to taste. Place slices of
French bread that have been sautéed in a little oil and margarine in the bottom of each soup bowl, place a piece of fish

on it, pour over the soup, and top with a spoonful of mayonnaise that's been mixed with a crushed clove of garlic.

## CARROT AND TARRAGON SOUP

2 oz margarine
1½ lb carrots, scraped and chopped
a medium potato, peeled and chopped
a medium onion, chopped
3 cups chicken broth
½ teaspoon (dried or fresh) tarragon
Salt

Melt the margarine and stir in the vegetables. Cover and cook for ten minutes. Add the broth and the seasonings, simmer for about twenty-five minutes, and put through a blender. Serve either hot or cold

## COLD CUCUMBER SOUP

2 tablespoons chopped onion
1 tablespoon safflower oil
1½ cups diced cucumber
¾ cup watercress
4 tablespoons finely diced raw potato
1½ cups chicken broth
2 sprigs parsley
½ teaspoon salt
Snipped chives

Cook the onion in the oil until transparent. Add the remaining ingredients and bring to a boil. Reduce the heat and simmer about fifteen minutes. When the potatoes are tender, puree and chill. Serve with chopped chives.

## SWEET CORN SOUP

1 lb tin of creamed sweet corn
3 cups chicken broth

1 *tablespoon sherry*
¼ *teaspoon sesame oil*
*Salt to taste*
1 *egg white, stiffly beaten*

Combine all ingredients except the egg white in a saucepan and bring to a boil. Simmer gently for about two minutes, then fold in the stiffly beaten egg white and serve immediately.

## DR DONG'S MAGIC MIXTURE

This is to be carried in a thermos, hot. It's fine for a football game, a winter outing or anything of that sort, but it is actually what Dr Dong takes to his office every day of his life. It's sustaining, perfect nourishment, and he makes it himself every morning.

Put a cup or so of left-over cooked rice in a blender, add a cooked vegetable such as carrots (this depends on your taste – I like onion and carrots) and a little cooked white fish or you can use breast of chicken. Add one and a half cups of water, and a little salt, and blend thoroughly. Put it in a pan, add another cup of water, and heat it to the boiling point. Then add about half a dessertspoon of safflower oil and put the mixture into the thermos. Dr Dong drinks a cup of this about every two hours while he's in his office; I think it explains how he maintains his backbreaking schedule. This concoction could very well be the answer for those who take their lunch to work.

## CHINESE EGGDROP SOUP

½ *tablespoon cornstarch*
2 *cups chicken broth*
1 *egg white*
1 *spring onion, chopped, top and all*
1 *teaspoon salt*

Dissolve the cornstarch in two tablespoons of the cold broth; heat the remaining broth to boiling and add the cornstarch mixture, stirring. Beat the egg white with a fork, and slowly pour into the broth. Add the salt, stir once lightly and remove from the heat; serve with spring onions sprinkled on top.

## SHELLFISH SOUP

1 *dessertspoon olive oil*
1 *dessertspoon safflower oil*
1 *large onion, chopped fine*
1 *clove garlic, crushed*
2 *carrots, chopped fine*
4 *cups chicken broth*
2¼ *cups concentrated fish stock*
4 *tablespoons dry vermouth*
½ *teaspoon basil*
½ *teaspoon thyme*
*A few threads of saffron*
2 *small tins clams (if available)*
1 *lb medium shrimp, shelled and deveined*
1 *dozen oysters*

Heat the olive and safflower oil, add the onion, garlic and carrots, and sauté till tender. Add the chicken broth, fish stock, vermouth, basil, thyme and saffron, and simmer for about half an hour. Let cool, and refrigerate for at least twenty-four hours. When ready to serve, reheat the broth to boiling, and add the clams, shrimp, and oysters. Cover. Reduce heat and simmer for about eight minutes. This will serve six generously – ask some friends in!

# 21

## Salads

### AVOCADO STUFFED WITH CHICKEN SALAD

Mix together: diced, cooked chicken breasts, diced celery and cucumber, chopped spring onion, and safflower mayonnaise. Serve in an avocado half on lettuce leaves.

### CELERY VICTOR

Scrape and trim celery stalks into uniform lengths, discarding the tougher parts. Cover with water, add three tablespoons soy sauce, and simmer till tender. Marinate in safflower oil and salt.

### CHEF'S SALAD BOWL

Wash and thoroughly dry crisp lettuce. Add a handful of small shrimp, some white meat of chicken cut in matchstick strips, some slivers of green pepper, a good amount of chopped celery and spring onion, and a hard-boiled egg white. Dress with oil, garlic salt and a little dill.

### CRAB AND RICE SALAD

½ lb fresh or tinned crabmeat
1 cup cooked, chilled rice
⅓ cup chopped celery
2 spring onions, chopped
2 tablespoons sliced water chestnuts

½ *teaspoon soy sauce*
3 *tablespoons mayonnaise*
*Lettuce leaves*

Mix together all the ingredients except the lettuce, and chill well. Serve in crisp lettuce nests.

## FISH ASPIC SALAD

2 *tablespoons unflavoured gelatine*
¾ *cup cold water*
1¼ *cups cold chicken broth*
1 *dessertspoon liquid from pimento-stuffed olives*
¾ *cup flaked cooked fish (sole, halibut, etc.)*
1 *tablespoon chopped pimento-stuffed olives*
*Lettuce and watercress*

Dissolve the gelatine in the water and cook over low heat for about five minutes, stirring constantly. Remove from the heat, add the chicken broth, olive liquid, and a pinch of salt, and chill till the mixture thickens slightly. Fold in the fish and chopped olives, turn into a mould, and chill until firm. Unmould on the lettuce.

## FISH SALAD

1 *lb firm white fish (such as turbot), poached, drained and chilled; or tinned tuna*
2 *tablespoons chopped onion*
2 *tablespoons chopped parsley*
1 *large bay leaf, finely crumbled*
*About 5 tablespoons olive oil*
*Salt to taste*
*Slivered celery*

Cut the fish into bite-sized pieces; marinate with dressing made from the onion, parsley, bay leaf, olive oil, and salt. Serve slivered celery on the side.

## ORGANIC SALAD

1½ *cups shredded cabbage*
1 *cup fresh bean sprouts*
¾ *cup shredded carrots*
1 *dessertspoon olive oil*
1½ *dessertspoons mayonnaise*
1 *dessertspoon maple syrup*
½ *dessertspoon crushed coriander*
½ *dessertspoon chopped spring onions*
*Salt to taste*
*Dash of garlic (optional)*

Mix all ingredients together and chill in refrigerator. This salad will keep for several days.


## SALADE NIÇOISE

*New potatoes, boiled whole in their jackets*
*Green beans, cooked crisp*
*Beetroots, cooked*
*Tuna (the best white obtainable)*
*Lettuce*
*Anchovies*
*Black olives*
½ *cup olive oil*
1 *clove garlic*
*A touch of dry mustard*
*A good dash of salt*

Chill the potatoes, beans, beetroots, and tuna, and arrange on a bed of lettuce in the desired proportions. Decorate with strips of anchovies and black olives. Crush olive oil, add mustard and salt, and pour over the salad.

## SPINACH-SHRIMP SALAD

Wash tender young spinach leaves and dry carefully. Add shrimp and chopped, hard-boiled egg whites. Toss lightly with safflower oil mixed with a little olive oil and seasoned with garlic salt.

## 22

## Spaghetti sauces

### SPAGHETTI A LA VONGOLE

4 *cloves of garlic, crushed (cut this amount down if you don't*
   *like garlic as much as I do)*
2 *tablespoons olive oil*
2 *lb tinned chopped clams (reserve the liquid)*
*A glass of white wine*
2 *oz margarine*
¾ *cup finely chopped fresh basil*

Cook the garlic briefly in the olive oil, add the liquid from
the clams and the wine, and simmer for at least half an hour.
Cook one pound of spaghetti in plenty of boiling salted water,
drain off most of the water and add the margarine. Add the
clams and basil to the reduced sauce, heat through, and
serve over the spaghetti.

### PESTO

1½ *cups fresh basil*
½ *cup olive oil*
1 *tablespoon pine nuts*
2 *cloves garlic, crushed*
1 *teaspoon salt*
1½ *tablespoons margarine (at room temperature)*

Grind the basil with the oil in a mortar until you have a

paste. Add the pine nuts and grind them into the paste. When it is all smooth, add the other ingredients. Prepare your spaghetti as before and pour the sauce over it just before serving.

**23**

# Fish

## BROCHETTE PROVENÇAL

1 *lb firm white fish (bass, sole, cod, flounder, etc.)*
8 *large prawns*
8 *scallops*
*Flour*
2 *egg whites, slightly beaten*
½ *teaspoon salt*
1 *dessertspoon safflower oil*

Cut the fish into eight pieces and arrange the seafood alternately on four skewers. Roll them in flour, then in a mixture of the egg whites, salt and oil. Sauté in safflower oil or barbecue over charcoal.

## FISH CREOLE

½ *lb any firm white fish fillets, fresh or frozen*
1 *tablespoon flour*
1 *dessertspoon margarine*
1 *dessertspoon safflower oil*
4 *tablespoons water*
4 *tablespoons sliced celery*
2 *tablespoons sliced spring onions with tops*
2 *tablespoons chopped green pepper*
1 *clove garlic, crushed*
¾ *cup white sauce*
1 *bay leaf*

¼ *teaspoon thyme*
1 *tablespoon chopped parsley*
*Hot, cooked rice*

Thaw the fish if frozen, and cut into one-inch pieces. Brown
the flour in the margarine and oil, remove from the heat, and
cool slightly. Add the water gradually and stir till blended.
Add everything else except the fish and rice, cover, and
simmer for twenty minutes or until the vegetables are tender.
Remove the bay leaf, add the fish, and simmer for ten
minutes longer or until the fish flakes easily. Serve on a bed
of rice.


## FISH STUFFED WITH HERBS

*Any firm white fish, 3 lb in weight – or a 3 lb section of a larger*
  *fish*
1 *dessertspoon Chervil*
1 *dessertspoon fresh tarragon (or ½ teaspoon dried tarragon)*
1 *teaspoon dried fennel*
2 *large stalks celery, cut in strips*
1 *onion, chopped fine*
*Several lettuce leaves*
¼ *lb mushrooms*
*A clove of garlic*
½ *cup of oil*
¼ *lb margarine*

Skin and clean the fish. Salt the inside and stuff with the
herbs, celery and onion. Put the fish in a baking dish and
cover with lettuce leaves that have been dipped in boiling
water. Chop the mushrooms quite finely, crush the garlic
and sauté them together in the oil and margarine. Pour the
result over the fish and bake for about half an hour, or
until the fish will flake easily. Remove it to a hot dish, reduce
the remaining juices somewhat and pour over the fish.

## FISH MARTIGUES

½ *onion, sliced*
2 *cloves garlic, crushed*
2 *anchovies, well rinsed in hot water*
2½ *lb any firm white fish*
*Salt*
⅔ *cup fish stock or water*
1 *tablespoon white wine*
1 *dessertspoon flour*
1 *olive oil dessertspoon*
1 *dessertspoon margarine*

Mix the onion, garlic and anchovies and place them in the bottom of an oiled baking dish. Place the fish on this bed, salt very lightly, moisten with the stock (or water) and wine, and bake at 350 degrees (gas No. 3½) for about twenty-five minutes. In another pan, blend the flour into the olive oil and brown slightly. After the fish has been removed to a serving dish, pour the juices from the baking dish into the flour-oil roux and beat with a wire whisk. Cook over low heat for a few minutes, beating, then beat in the margarine and serve with the fish.

## COD (OR HADDOCK) WITH MUSHROOMS

¾ *cup chopped celery*
1 *tablespoon chopped chives*
¾ *cup chicken broth*
1 *lb cod or haddock fillets*
*Salt*
*Paprika*
4 *tablespoons sliced mushrooms*
2 *teaspoons margarine*

Cook the celery and chives in the chicken broth for about 5 minutes, then puree in a blender. Place the fish fillets in an oiled baking dish, sprinkle with a little salt and paprika, pour over the celery mixture, and arrange the mushrooms over all. Dot with the margarine and bake at 400 degrees (gas No. 5) for about a quarter of an hour.

## SOLE OR (FLOUNDER) BONNE FEMME

¼ *lb fresh mushrooms, chopped*
1 *dessertspoon minced shallot*
1½ *tablespoons minced parsley*
*Salt to taste*
1½ *lb sole (or flounder) fillets*
1 *cup court bouillon*
*Margarine*
*Parsley*

Mix together the mushrooms, shallot and parsley, and spread on the bottom of a margarined shallow casserole or pan. Salt the fillets, arrange them on the mushrooms, and pour the court bouillon over all. Cook for about twenty minutes in a 350-degree oven (gas No. 3½). Remove the fillets, keeping them warm while you reduce the sauce to about three-quarter cup. Add a tablespoon of margarine and pour over the sole. Garnish with sprigs of parsley and serve.

## SOLE OR FLOUNDER CHINOISE

It is simple Chinese-style cooking at its best, delicious and easy to prepare.

Take fillets of sole or flounder, the number depending on their size, and poach them in a small amount of water into which you've sliced thinly some fresh ginger root. They will only need to poach for about three or four minutes; test with a fork for flaking. Remove the fish from the water, to a serving dish and sprinkle with chopped spring onions and more thin slices of ginger root as a garnish. Heat some sesame oil and pour it and a small amount of soy sauce over the fish and serve.

## BAKED HADDOCK OR HALIBUT

Ask your fishmonger to bone a nice piece of haddock or halibut. Lay the fish in an ovenproof dish, with chopped onions, parsley, and green pepper, between the two pieces. Pour a little safflower oil over and around the fish, and bake in a preheated 350-degree oven (gas No. 3½) for about forty minutes for two to three pounds, one and a half hours for a whole fish. Baste from time to time with fish stock. If you like, you can add a handful of shrimp or prawns about ten minutes before it's done.

## COQUILLES ST JACQUES

1 *lb scallops*
1 *pt water with small bay leaf, pinch thyme, few sprigs parsley*
1 *tablespoon chopped parsley*
*Bunch spring onions, chopped*
1½ *oz margarine*
*Salt*
½ *oz flour*
*Breadcrumbs*

Wash and drain the scallops. If large cut into pieces; if small leave whole. Simmer in the water till tender, about five or six minutes. Remove with a slotted spoon, set aside, and boil the water rapidly till reduced almost by half. If you're a garlic lover, crush in two cloves garlic. Add the spring onions and parsley; simmer in the liquid ten minutes. Make a *roux* of the flour and margarine; gradually add the liquid; salt to taste. After you have a nice creamy sauce, stir in the scallops, place them in baking shells, top with breadcrumbs, dot with margarine, and slide under the grill until nicely browned.

## POACHED SALMON WITH GREEN MAYONNAISE

This can be done either with a large fillet of salmon or the desired number of salmon steaks. Bring to a simmer in a shallow pan, enough court bouillon to cover the fish, and slide the salmon in. Maintain the heat evenly at a simmer; watch the salmon carefully because it cooks quickly and is best when a trifle underdone. Lift from the bouillon with a slotted spoon, drain carefully and place on a heated platter.

Serve with the following sauce: Drop a handful of spinach leaves, a small handful of watercress leaves and a small handful of parsley sprigs in boiling water for just a minute. Drain well in paper towels, and chop very, very fine. Stir into one and a half cups of safflower mayonnaise.

## SALMON EN CROUTE

This is one of my favourites. It's impressive, not hard to do, and absolutely delicious. An ideal way to use a whole salmon is to entertain twice with it. I bake it the first time, serving only the top half – in other words, serving off the bone. Then, depending on when I plan to use the other half, I either freeze it or refrigerate it. When I'm ready to use it, I carefully remove the bone – the spine will usually come away in one piece when it's cold – and the skin. You can however, start out with a large fillet, or even a small whole fish, which you can bone after cooking. In any case, we now have a good-sized piece of cooked salmon.

Make a pastry as for Chicken Pie (see page 203); when chilled, divide it in half. Roll out half the pastry in the shape of and slightly larger than the salmon. Place the piece of pastry on an ovenproof dish and lay the fish carefully on it. (It takes a bit of doing not to break it, but if you do, you can piece it together.) Now spread on the fish half a cup of rice cooked in fish stock with a little tarragon. Sprinkle this with chopped hard-boiled egg whites and chopped parsley. Roll out the other half of the pastry, allowing enough extra for the mound of the fish, and place on top. Wet the edges with a pastry brush and crimp with a fork. Make one or two slits in the top, and pour in a large amount of melted margarine – two ounces for a good-sized fish. Bake in a preheated 400-degree oven (gas No. 5) until the pastry is lightly browned.

To serve, slice down through the layers of rice and fish,

and serve with mayonnaise thinned down with a little fish
stock and a tiny bit of white wine.


## SHISH KEBAB

*Scallops and/or large prawns or scampi*
*Green peppers, cut in hunks*
*Quartered onions*
*Large whole mushrooms*
*Olive oil*
*A garlic clove, crushed*
*A bay leaf*
*Tarragon*
*Oregano*

Allow about four scallops and/or prawns per person.
Marinate the fish and vegetables in the olive oil, garlic, bay
leaf and about a teaspoon each tarragon and oregano.
Thread on skewers and barbecue or grill.


## BAKED SHRIMP

*2½ tablespoons margarine*
*2½ tablespoons flour*
*1½ cups chicken broth*
*1 teaspoon salt*
*Few dessertspoons dry sherry*
*2¼ cups hot, cooked rice*
*4 tablespoons chopped parsley*
*4 tablespoons sliced spring onions, tops and all*
*2 cups cooked shrimp*

Melt the margarine, and add the flour to make a roux.
Slowly add the chicken broth, and stir till the sauce thickens.
Add the remaining ingredients and turn into a shallow baking
dish. Bake about twenty minutes in a 350-degree oven (gas
No. 3½).

## POACHED SOLE CHAUDFROID

*4 even-sized sole fillets (you might substitute flounder, although
the flavour is not quite so delicate)*
*Court bouillon flavoured with tarragon*
*1 tablespoon gelatine*
*1½ cups safflower mayonnaise*
*Watercress*

Cover the sole with the court bouillon; reduce the heat and
simmer very gently until nearly done. At this point remove the
pan from the stove and let the sole finish cooking in the broth.
Then let the broth cool, carefully remove the sole and put it
on a serving dish. Soften the gelatine in eight tablespoons
of the broth; dissolve over hot water. Blend in the safflower
mayonnaise, and chill. When the mayonnaise mixture is
thickened, but not gelled, pour over the fish to mask it. This
thickening process should take about half an hour. Watch it
carefully – once it gells, you've had it! Remove the fish from
the refrigerator about half an hour ahead of serving so it
won't be too cold. Garnish with watercress.

## SOLE, FLOUNDER OR SEA BREAM MEUNIÈRE

*A tablespoon safflower oil*
*A tablespoon margarine*
*4 small fillets of sole, flounder or sea bream*
*Flour*
*Salt*
*Chopped parsley*

Heat the oil and margarine in a heavy frying pan, dust the
fillets with flour, salt lightly, and sauté in the hot oil and
margarine till lightly browned, turning once. (About two
minutes to a side should be enough.) Transfer to a hot dish,
add the chopped parsley to the oil and margarine in the pan,
stir, and pour over the fish.

## FISH CASSEROLE I

2 oz margarine
1 smallish onion, chopped
1 tablespoon flour
1¼ cups fish stock
1 lb of any firm white fish
Breadcrumbs

Melt the margarine and sauté the onion. Gradually work in
the flour to make a smooth mixture; add the fish stock
gradually and stir till thick. Pour this over the fish in a
shallow casserole and top with breadcrumbs. Bake in a 350-
degree oven (gas No. 3½) for twenty minutes.

## FISH CASSEROLE II

½ onion, chopped
¼ green pepper, sliced thin
1 dessertspoon safflower oil
1 dessertspoon margarine
1 dessertspoon flour
¾ cup chicken broth
Heaped dessertspoon sliced tinned pimentos
Salt
½ lb of any firm white fish
Paprika

Sauté the onion and green pepper in the oil and margarine.
Pull them to one side of the pan, work the flour into the
remaining oil and margarine, and simmer, stirring, for one
or two minutes. Slowly add the broth and stir till thickened
and creamy. Add the pimentos, a little salt, and pour the
sauce over the fish in a shallow baking dish. Sprinkle with a
few dashes of paprika and bake in a 350-degree oven (gas No.
3½) for twenty minutes.

## FISH PIE

2 *carrots, diced*
1 *large potato, diced*
1 *large onion, chopped*
½ *lb of any firm white fish*
⅔ *cup white sauce (see recipe for Fish Surprise, page 200)*
*Biscuit dough (see below)*

Cook the vegetables in a little boiling water till just tender; drain. Cook the fish for about ten minutes in water, stock or a court bouillon. Drain and flake it, and mix with the vegetables and white sauce in an oiled baking dish. Cover with biscuit dough and bake for twenty minutes at 375 degrees (gas No. 4).

*Pastry*

Sift ¾ cup of flour with 1½ teaspoons of baking powder; cut in a tablespoon of margarine and add about ¼ cup of water. Mix well and add a little more water if necessary. Turn out on a lightly floured board and form into a smooth ball; roll out to a ¼-inch thickness and cover the fish with it.

## FISH SOUFFLÉ

1 *dessertspoon flour*
1 *dessertspoon margarine*
10 *tablespoons water*
4 *tablespoons soft breadcrumbs*
½ *lb of any firm white fish*
1 *teaspoon chopped parsley*
1 *teaspoon chopped chives*
1 *teaspoon onion juice*
*Salt*
3 *egg whites, well beaten*

Make a cream sauce by blending the flour with the margarine, cooking and stirring till creamy smooth. Add the water slowly and stir, cooking till smooth. Add the breadcrumbs and continue cooking for a few minutes, then add the rest of the ingredients and mix well. Lastly, fold in the egg whites and bake in a 400-degree (gas No. 5) oven for about twenty-five minutes. Chopped sautéed mushrooms are good served with this dish.

## FISH SURPRISE

1 *onion, finely chopped*
1 *dessertspoon safflower oil*
1½ *tablespoons margarine*
1 *tablespoon flour*
1½ *cups chicken broth*
1 *lb of any firm white fish*
*Small packet potato crisps, crumbled*

Brown the onion in the oil and a dessertspoon of the margarine. Make a white sauce by mixing one tablespoon flour with the rest of the margarine, cooking for a minute or two, and gradually adding the chicken broth. Cook the fish as for Fish Pie, flake it and put in layers in a baking dish, alternating the fish, white sauce and a small packet of crumbled potato crisps. Bake for twenty minutes at 350 degrees (gas No. 3½).

# Chicken

## BAKED CHICKEN WITH HERBS

6 *chicken breasts*
2½ *tablespoons olive oil and safflower oil, mixed half and half*
½ *teaspoon each thyme, basil and marjoram*
1 *dessertspoon fresh-cut chives*
*Flour*
*Salt*
¾ *cup water*
1 *dessertspoon minced parsley*

Wipe the chicken breasts with a damp cloth. Place in a bowl and pour 1½ tablespoons of oil over them; sprinkle with the mixed herbs and chives. Cover, and let stand in the refrigerator for three or four hours. Lift the chicken from the marinade, dust lightly with flour, and brown for a quarter of an hour in the rest of the oil. Arrange the breasts in one layer in a large, shallow casserole; salt lightly. Mix the marinade remaining in the bowl with the water; add the parsley to it and pour this over the chicken. Cover and bake in a 375-degree oven (gas No. 4) for half an hour. Uncover periodically to see if the chicken is done; baste frequently with the marinade in the casserole.

## CHICKEN BREASTS CHINOISE

Place two skinned chicken breasts in a shallow pan. Mix a tablespoon of soy sauce with a tablespoon of sesame oil, ½ teaspoon of salt and ¼ teaspoon of ginger. Brush the chicken with this mixture and bake uncovered for about forty-five minutes at 350 degrees (gas No. 3½).

## CHICKEN BREASTS MARY ELIZABETH

2 *chicken breasts, skinned and boned*
1 *egg white, slightly beaten*
¾ *cup breadcrumbs*
*Safflower oil*
¾ *cup chicken broth*
1 *dessertspoon cornstarch*
*Curry powder*
*Salt*

Dip the chicken in the egg white, then roll in the bread-crumbs. Sauté in about ¼ inch of safflower oil. Place in a baking dish, pour over the chicken broth thickened with the cornstarch and seasoned with a pinch of curry powder and salt. Bake for twenty minutes in a 350-degree oven (gas No. 3½).

## CHICKEN IN A WOK

A wok is a Chinese cooking utensil, a metal pan shaped like a bowl that holds heat uniformly over its surface and cooks quickly and evenly. It isn't essential; you can prepare this in a deep frying pan. But woks are good for this sort of cooking and fun to use.

1 *large chicken breast, boned and cut in strips*
½ *teaspoon powdered ginger*
¼ *teaspoon salt*
*Dash paprika*
1 *dessertspoon safflower oil*
6 *tablespoons diagonally sliced celery*
2 *tablespoons sliced green pepper*
2 *tablespoons chopped spring onion*
1 *cup chicken broth*

1 *dessertspoon soy sauce*
½ *dessertspoon cornstarch mixed with a little cold water*

Toss the chicken in the ginger, salt and paprika. Heat the oil in the wok and sauté the chicken for about five minutes, stirring frequently. Push the chicken aside, add the vegetables, and cook for about five minutes longer, stirring frequently. Add the broth and the soy sauce, cover and cook on low heat for another five minutes. Stir in the cornstarch, cook till the sauce thickens slightly, and serve.

## CHICKEN PIE

*Pastry:*
3 *oz margarine*
¾ *cup flour*
Large pinch salt
1 *to* 1½ *tablespoons cold water*
An egg white, slightly beaten

Break the margarine up into bits and add to the dry ingredients. Mix with your hands till blended, and add the egg white and enough water to allow you to make the dough into a ball. Refrigerate for an hour before rolling out. The egg white is for later.

*Filling:*

6 *or* 8 *chicken breasts (skinned)*
2½ *pints chicken broth*
About 10 *small white pickling onions*
2 *carrots, scraped and sliced lengthwise*
¼ *lb mushrooms*
2½ *tablespoons flour*
2 *oz margarine*
¼ *teaspoon salt*
1 *or* 2 *dozen oysters (optional)*

Cover the chicken with the broth, bring to the boil and simmer till tender. Remove the chicken and skim any scum from the surface of the broth. Add the onions and carrots and simmer for ten minutes; add the mushrooms and cook until all the vegetables are tender. Remove them from the broth. While they are cooking, remove the chicken meat from the bones, cutting it into serving-sized pieces. Make a cream sauce of the flour, margarine and a little less than half the broth. Salt, mix with the chicken and vegetables and pour into a baking dish. Top with the pastry, make a few slits for steam, brush with the egg white, and bake for forty-five minutes at 350 degrees (gas No. 3½). The addition of oysters to this pie makes a delightful combination of flavours.

## CHICKEN WITH BROCCOLI

Slightly undercook a bunch of broccoli, and lay it in the bottom of a casserole. Poach three boned chicken breasts in just enough water to barely cover them, reserving half a pint of the resulting broth. Brown the breasts in a little oil and margarine, place them on the broccoli, and pour over them a sauce made from mixing the chicken broth with four table-spoons of safflower mayonnaise, half a teaspoon of coriander and a very slight pinch of curry powder. Bake for about fifteen or twenty minutes at 350 degrees (gas No. 3½).

## DR DONG'S CHICKEN

Wash and dry one whole roasting chicken and salt it lightly. Make a paste of a tablespoon each of brown sugar and thick soy sauce. (If you cannot find the thick soy sauce, use the regular, but check the label carefully for MSG and other additives.) Cover the chicken with about half the paste and put into the oven on a rack. Cook for half an hour at 400 degrees (gas No. 5). Baste with the remaining sugar and soy sauce, adding a tablespoon of vegetable oil to the mixture. This will prevent the skin from drying out. You might also add a loose foil cover at this time to keep the skin from getting too dark. Decrease the oven heat to 375 degrees (gas No. 4) and continue to bake for another half an hour. To test if it is done, cut into the thickest part of the chicken; it should not be pink.

## TURKEY WITH OYSTER STUFFING

Everyone seems to have a best way to cook a turkey. I've experimented with everything from precooking and reheating to baking it in one of my husband's green Marine T-shirts. Currently I cook it loosely covered in foil until the final browning, and baste it frequently. My oyster dressing is very simple: For an average-sized turkey, say ten to twelve pounds, I use two dozen oysters. Cut them up if they're large, saving the juice. Add about 4½ cups of cubed, slightly stale bread, 1½ cups of minced celery, ¾ cup of minced onion and 4 oz of melted margarine, and mix it all together with the oyster juice. Stuff the turkey and secure it firmly. Rub the outside of the bird with a mixture of safflower oil and margarine. Roast uncovered at 325 degrees (gas No. 3) for fifteen to eighteen minutes per pound. The turkey is done when the leg moves easily. If it browns too fast, cover it with a tent of foil.

## TURKEY WITH TUNA

(*Start the day before*)

4 *lb of turkey breast*
*A large onion, chopped*
2 *stalks celery, chopped*
2 *cloves garlic, crushed*
*A carrot, chopped*
*An 8-oz tin white tuna (in oil)*
4 *pints chicken broth*
¾ *cup white wine*
½ *teaspoon thyme*
*A tube of anchovy paste*
*Capers*
2¼ *cups safflower oil mayonnaise*
1½ *cups rice (packeted, not wild)*

*1½ tablespoons safflower oil*
*¾ cup parsley, finely chopped*

Remove any fat from the turkey and place it breast down in a large heavy pan that has a cover. Add all the other ingredients except the last five. There should be enough liquid to cover the meat; if not add more broth or water. Bring to the boil, reduce the heat, cover the pan with wax paper and the lid, and simmer till turkey is tender – about two hours. Place covered pan in refrigerator over night.

The following day remove the breast, wrap it in foil and return to refrigerator. Over high heat reduce the liquid to about three cups; strain through a fine sieve. Refrigerate. When cold, skim off fat from top. Put the mayonnaise in a bowl and gradually beat in enough of the broth to make a thick smooth sauce. Carve the turkey in thin uniform slices. Cook the rice; add the safflower oil, then the parsley. Serve the turkey on a bed of the rice, masking the meat with the sauce. Garnish with capers. Serve the remaining sauce in a bowl.

The left-overs from this dish will make a great dinner for the next night. You'll have some of the sauce left, as there is quite a lot. Cook some spaghetti, cut the remaining turkey into small pieces and add to the hot sauce. Pour it over spaghetti and serve.

## CREAMED CABBAGE

Pour boiling water over a small head of shredded cabbage and allow to cook for three minutes. Drain the cabbage, hold it under cold running water, and drain it again. Sauté 1½ tablespoons of minced onion in a dessertspoon of margarine until soft, add the cabbage, 4 tablespoons of safflower mayonnaise, ¼ teaspoon of dill and salt to taste. Simmer, stirring and tossing, for about three minutes.

## GADO GADO

A Dutch friend of mine serves this delicious Indonesian vegetable dish for lunch. The combination of ingredients is such that one need serve nothing else; it's a complete meal.

Cut up and steam 4 or 5 vegetables such as carrots, bean sprouts, brussels sprouts, green beans and cabbage. (The bean sprouts are the only essential.) They should be crisply undercooked. Arrange them in neat sections in a serving dish and allow them to cool to room temperature. Make a sauce of peanut butter – the crunchy kind – and water. It should be about the consistency of mayonnaise. Put it on the stove and stir till smooth, then add a crushed clove of garlic, a little cayenne (just a dash), soy sauce to taste and some finely minced onion. Serve the sauce lukewarm in a separate bowl. Prawn crackers, available in Chinese delicatessens, are delicious served with this dish.

## POLENTA

1½ *cups water*
4 *tablespoons cornmeal*
1 *tablespoon margarine*

Bring the water to a boil, slowly add the cornmeal and boil for five minutes. Add the margarine, place in a baking dish and bake for about half an hour in a 350-degree oven (gas No. 3½).

## DOLLAR POTATOES

Choose long, not round, baking potatoes. Holding the potato firmly in one hand, slice it thinly across the narrow way, making coin-like discs. Keeping the potato slices together so the potato is in its original shape, place in a pan where it will fit snugly and not fall apart. (If necessary pad around it with foil.) Brush well with margarine and bake for an hour at 400 degrees (gas No. 5), or until crisp and done.

## RICE PILAF WITH VEGETABLES

¼ *lb margarine*
*A small aubergine, peeled and dried*
*A small courgette, diced*
2 *large mushrooms, sliced*
*A clove garlic, crushed*
*A small tin pimentos, minced*
*A teaspoon salt*
½ *lb rice*
¾ *pint chicken broth*

Melt the margarine in a saucepan, add everything except the rice and broth and sauté lightly. Add the broth, bring to a boil, add the rice. Cover tightly and cook over low heat for about half an hour.

## CREAMED SPINACH

*A packet of frozen chopped spinach*
*4 tablespoons safflower mayonnaise*
*Pinch nutmeg*
*Dash salt*

This is one of the few times I use a frozen vegetable for convenience. (The spinach is all chopped and easy to use, but you may very well prefer to cook and chop fresh spinach.) Without adding any water, cook the spinach in a covered pan only till defrosted and very hot. Gradually stir in the mayonnaise over very low heat. Add a pinch of nutmeg, a dash of salt, stir till very hot and smooth, and serve at once.

## SPINACH-STUFFED MUSHROOM CAPS

*½ packet frozen spinach*
*1 dessertspoon margarine*
*1 dessertspoon flour*
*Pinch nutmeg*
*Salt to taste*
*4 large mushrooms, washed and peeled (if necessary)*

Cook the spinach slightly, saving the juice. Melt the margarine and stir in the flour to make a roux. Gradually add enough spinach water to make a thick sauce, about ½ cup. Add the nutmeg and salt, then mix with the spinach. Stuff the mushroom caps and bake in a 350-degree oven (gas No. 3½) until the mushrooms are done – around seven to ten minutes.

## VEGETABLE PANCAKES

*The Pancakes:*

*1 cup flour*
*1 dessertspoon sugar*
*1 teaspoon baking powder*
*½ teaspoon salt*

1 *egg white*
¾ *cup of water*
1 *tablespoon safflower oil*

*The Filling:*

*Sliced mushrooms*
*Chopped spring onions*
*Chopped green peppers*
*Bean sprouts*
*A very ripe avocado, peeled and mashed*
*A clove of garlic, crushed*
½ *tablespoon very finely chopped onion*
*A drop of Tabasco sauce*

Sift the dry ingredients together; beat the egg white lightly
and add the other wet ingredients and mix thoroughly.
Combine the wet and dry ingredients and stir just enough to
mix together. The batter should be lumpy.

For the filling, make a guacamole out of the avocado,
garlic, onion and Tabasco. Sauté the mushrooms or serve
them raw, as desired.

## VEGETABLES WITH HERBS

2 *slices aubergine*
*A small courgette*
*A green pepper*
*A small onion*
*Olive oil*
*Safflower oil*
*Breadcrumbs*
*A tablespoon of chopped parsley*
*A clove of garlic, crushed*
½ *teaspoon crumbled basil*
*Rosemary*
*Sage*
*Salt*

Slice the vegetables and moisten them with olive and

safflower oil, mixed. Lay them in a baking pan and top with
the breadcrumbs mixed with the parsley, garlic, basil, a
large pinch each of rosemary and sage, and $\frac{1}{4}$ teaspoon of
salt. Bake in a 350-degree oven (gas No. $3\frac{1}{2}$) till crisply
tender. Allow to cool before serving.


## BRAISED COURGETTES

Slice the courgettes on the diagonal, about half an inch
thick, and place in a heavy pan with a pat of margarine. Melt
the margarine, add salt and cover. Braise over very low heat
till tender but not soft – ten minutes should be enough.


## COURGETTE FRITATA

3 or 4 courgettes, chopped
A smallish onion, chopped
A clove of garlic, crushed
A tablespoon of olive oil
3 egg whites
A tablespoon of flour
Salt
Nutmeg

Sauté the vegetables and garlic lightly in the olive oil. Beat
the egg whites until frothy; add the flour, salt and a little
nutmeg. Mix with the vegetables and pour into a small,
shallow baking dish. Bake until the eggs are set – about
eight minutes in a 350-degree oven (gas No. $3\frac{1}{2}$).


## RATATOUILLE

$\frac{3}{4}$ lb marrow
3 large cloves of garlic, crushed
6 tablespoons olive oil
1 teaspoon cumin seeds, crushed
Half an aubergine
1 teaspoon oregano
3 onions, sliced thin

*2 green peppers, seeded and cut into strips*
*½ teaspoon marjoram*
*½ teaspoon dill*
*Salt*

Peel the aubergine, cut it into small cubes, salt it and let it stand for a half hour or so. Cube the marrow and put it in the bottom of an oiled casserole. To this layer add salt, one clove garlic, two tablespoons of the oil and the cumin seeds. Rinse and dry the aubergine, put it in the casserole and to this layer add salt, another clove of garlic, and the oregano. Now add the onions and green peppers, the rest of the garlic and oil, the marjoram and the dill. Cover and bake in a 350-degree oven (gas No. 3½) for an hour.

# Desserts

## DR DONG'S BASIC RICE PUDDING

4 *pints water*
1½ *cups uncooked rice*

Thoroughly wash the rice until the water runs clear. This is very important! Put the rice in a blender and add about a cup of cold water. Blend on the medium and then on the highest speed four times. The mixture will be milky and pulverised. Meanwhile, bring three pints of water to a rapid boil in a heavy container. Add the contents of the blender *very slowly*, stirring constantly with a serrated spoon. It will thicken almost immediately. Don't be afraid of this consistency; it will smooth out during the boiling. Boil for about twenty-five minutes, stirring occasionally, and if the mixture seems too lumpy use your whisk a few times while cooking. Pour into a bowl and chill. This mixture may be used as a cereal, a thickening agent for soups, with fish, or as a pudding with the addition of brown sugar or honey. Covered, the pudding will keep well in the refrigerator.

## WALNUT DESSERT

⅔ *cup sugar*
*A cup of light syrup*
¼ *lb of margarine, melted*
*A teaspoon of vanilla*
4 *egg whites*
1¼ *cups walnuts*

Beat the sugar, syrup, margarine and vanilla together; add the beaten egg whites and nuts and turn into an oiled eight-inch baking tin. Bake in a 375-degree oven (gas No. 4) for thirty-five to forty minutes.

## VANILLA SOUFFLÉ

2 oz margarine
1 oz flour
A cup of water
¼ lb castor sugar
A teaspoon of vanilla
¼ teaspoon almond extract
4 egg whites
Icing sugar
1 oz toasted chopped almonds

Make a white sauce of the margarine, flour and water; stir in the castor sugar and flavourings. Fold in the stiffly beaten egg whites, turn into an oiled soufflé dish and sprinkle with the icing sugar. Place in a pan of hot water and bake in a 350-degree oven (gas No. 3½) for about fifty-five minutes, or till firm. Sprinkle with the almonds and serve immediately.

## ANGEL CREAM

5 egg whites
2 oz castor sugar
A teaspoon of vanilla
2 oz grated almonds

Beat the egg whites till stiff, add two-thirds of the sugar and then gently fold in the remainder. Add the vanilla and gently fold in the almonds (these can be grated in a blender). Angel Cream should be served very cold, so since it must be done at the last minute (or the egg whites will separate), keep the ingredients in the refrigerator until ready to use. It only takes a few minutes to do so, and it is delicious.

## ZABAGLIONE

1 *envelope unflavoured gelatine*
2 *oz sugar*
*Salt*
*A cup of cold water.*
1½ *tablespoons Marsala wine*
2 *egg whites*

Melt the gelatine in some of the cold water, place over low heat and stir for about three minutes. Remove from heat and stir in the sugar, salt, remaining water and wine. Chill until the mixture is slightly thickened. Beat egg whites until stiff, then as you add the sugar mixture continue beating until it becomes very light, frothy and has doubled in volume. Chill until set.

## PUMPKIN CHIFFON PIE

*Crust:*
1¼ *cups finely ground Brazil nuts*
1½ *tablespoons sugar*

*Filling:*
1 *dessertspoon unflavoured gelatine*
½ *pint cold water*
1½ *cups cooked pumpkin*
4 *tablespoons sugar*
1¼ *teaspoons salt*
1 *teaspoon cinnamon*
½ *teaspoon ginger*
2 *egg whites*
2 *tablespoons shredded, toasted Brazil nuts*

For the crust, combine the ground Brazil nuts with the sugar and line an eight-inch pie dish. For the filling, soften the gelatine in half the cold water. Combine the pumpkin, half the sugar, salt, spices and remaining water; cook over boiling water for five minutes, stirring constantly. Stir in the softened gelatine until it is dissolved. Chill until slightly thickened. Then gradually beat the remaining sugar into the stiffly beaten egg whites and fold into the thickened pumpkin–gelatine mixture. Pour the filling on the crust mixture in the pie plate and top with the shredded nuts. Chill until firm.

## ANGEL FOOD CAKE

½ lb sugar
¼ pint water
¾ cup egg whites
1 teaspoon almond extract
3 oz flour
¼ teaspoon salt
1 teaspoon cream of tartar

Boil the sugar and water together until a thread forms when a spoon is dipped into it. Beat the egg whites until stiff; gradually beat in the sugar mixture, then add the almond extract and beat until cooled. Mix and sift the flour and other dry ingredients several times; then gradually fold in the beaten egg-white mixture. Bake in an ungreased cake-tin at 275 degrees (gas No. 1) for half an hour, then at 375 degrees (gas No. 4) until the cake springs back when pressed with a finger – about seven to ten minutes.

## CARROT CAKE

6 oz margarine
¾ lb sugar
4 egg whites
1 teaspoon ground cinnamon
½ teaspoon nutmeg
1¼ cups finely grated carrots
½ cup finely chopped toasted walnuts
1¾ cups sifted all-purpose flour
3 teaspoons baking powder
½ teaspoon salt
5–6 tablespoons warm water

Beat the softened margarine and sugar until light and fluffy, then beat in the egg whites and spices. Stir in the carrots and nuts. Sift the dry ingredients and add to the mixture alternately with the water. (Do not beat the flour mixture in, but rather fold it in till it is moistened.) Turn into an oiled and floured baking tin, and bake in a preheated 350-degree oven (gas No. 3½) for thirty-five minutes or until the cake springs back when pressed lightly in the centre. Cool on a cake rack.

## MAYONNAISE CAKE

1 *teaspoon baking soda*
4 *tablespoons chopped walnuts*
4 *tablespoons chopped almonds*
¾ *cup boiling water*
¼ *cup sugar*
5 *oz flour*
1 *teaspoon cinnamon*
¾ *cup safflower mayonnaise*

Add the soda to the nuts and pour the boiling water over them. Let cool. Mix the sugar, flour and cinnamon with the mayonnaise, combine with the nuts, and bake in a nine-inch tin for about half an hour at 350 degrees (gas No. 3½).

## ALMOND OATMEAL COOKIES

6 *oz margarine*
¾ *cup brown sugar*
4 *tablespoons water*
*A generous teaspoon of almond flavouring*
3 *oz flour*
½ *teaspoon baking soda*
1 *teaspoon salt*
1½ *cups Quick Quaker Oats*
4 *tablespoons finely chopped blanched almonds*

Mix the margarine, sugar, water and almond flavouring and beat till smooth. Sift the dry ingredients together and add to

the creamy mixture. Add the Quaker Oats and almonds.
Drop by the teaspoonful on to greased baking sheets and
press down slightly. Bake for fourteen minutes at 350
degrees (gas No. 3½).

## ITALIAN ANISE COOKIES

10 *oz sifted unbleached flour*
¼ *lb sugar*
1 *dessertspoon baking powder*
1½ *teaspoons salt*
4 *egg whites*
2 *to* 3 *teaspoons crushed anise seeds*
¾ *cup chopped roasted almonds*

Sift the flour with the sugar, baking powder and salt. Beat
the egg whites slightly with a fork; mix in the anise seeds and
flour mixture to make a soft dough. Divide in half. Roll each
half into a 10 × 8-inch rectangle. Sprinkle with the almonds
and roll up as for a swiss roll, starting from the ten-inch side.
Slide on to a greased baking sheet and flatten to about an
inch in height. Bake at 350 degrees (gas No. 3½) for twenty
to twenty-five minutes or until lightly browned. Cool slightly
and slice into ½-inch pieces; return the slices to the baking
sheet and toast in a 350-degree oven (gas No. 3½) for four
or five minutes.

## MACAROONS

6 *egg whites*
½ *teaspoon salt*
6 *oz sugar*
6 *or* 7 *oz blanched almonds*
2 *tablespoons white cornmeal or matzo meal*
½ *teaspoon rum flavouring*

Beat the egg whites and salt until fairly stiff; then add the
sugar slowly, continuing to beat until the egg whites form
firm peaks. Grind the almonds in a blender until very fine

and fork into the egg whites. Add the cornmeal and rum
flavouring and drop the mixture by teaspoons on to an oiled
baking sheet. Flatten slightly with a spoon and bake in a
350-degree oven (gas No. 3½) for about twenty minutes. Cool
slightly before removing from the sheet; cool further on a
rack.


## PFEFFER NUTS

¾ *cup unblanched almonds*
6 *oz unsifted flour*
1 *teaspoon baking soda*
4 *tablespoons dark syrup*
¼ *lb margarine*
6 *oz sugar*
1½ *teaspoons cinnamon*
½ *teaspoon nutmeg*
¼ *teaspoon cloves*
¼ *teaspoon salt*
1 *egg white*
*Icing sugar*

Grind the almonds coarsely in a blender; mix with the
unsifted flour and baking soda. Combine all the rest of the
ingredients except the egg white and icing sugar in a saucepan and heat, stirring, until the margarine melts. Cool
slightly, mix in the egg white and gradually beat in the
almond mixture. Chill the dough if it is too soft to handle,
then shape it into balls about the size of walnuts. Bake the
balls on an ungreased baking sheet in a 375-degree oven (gas
No. 4) for fifteen to twenty minutes, checking to make sure
they don't get too brown on the bottom. Shake the cookies,
while still warm, a few at a time, in a bag of icing sugar.


## SESAME SEED COOKIES

2 *oz shredded coconut*
¾ *cup sesame seeds*
⅔ *cup corn oil*

¾ *cup brown sugar*
1½ *cups flour*
½ *teaspoon baking soda*
1 *teaspoon baking powder*
½ *teaspoon salt*
*Vanilla or almond extract (whichever you prefer)*

Spread the coconut and sesame seeds on a baking sheet and toast them lightly. Cream the oil and sugar, and gradually sift in the dry ingredients. Add the vanilla or almond extract, and mix in the coconut and sesame seeds. Drop by the teaspoonful on to an oiled baking sheet and bake for twelve minutes at 350 degrees (gas No. 3½).

# Selected bibliography for the medical section

## Books

ABERCROMBIE, M., C. J. HICKMAN AND M. L. JOHNSON. *A Dictionary of Biology*. Penguin Books, Baltimore, 1964 and Harmondsworth, 1969.

ADAMS, JOHN CRAWFORD. *Arthritis and Back Pain*. University Park Press, Baltimore, 1972 and Medical and Technical Publishing, 1972.

ANATOMICAL SCIENCES TRAINING COMMITTEE OF THE NATIONAL INSTITUTE OF GENERAL MEDICAL SCIENCES. *Cellular Aspects of Immune Reaction*. National Institutes of Health, Bethesda, Md., 1967.

ASCHNER, BERNARD, M.D. *Arthritis Can Be Cured*. The Julian Press, Inc., New York, 1957.

BARNES, C. G., et al. (editors). *Clinical Rheumatology*. J. B. Lippincott Co., Philadelphia, 1970.

BEACH, FRANK A. *Hormones and Behavior*. Paul B. Hoeber, Inc., New York, 1948.

BEECHER, HENRY K. *Measurement of Subjective Responses: Quantitative Effects of Drugs*. Oxford University Press, New York, 1959.

BICKNELL, FRANKLIN AND FREDERICK PRESCOTT. *The American and His Food*. University of Chicago Press, Chicago, 1941.

BLAND, JOHN H., M.D. *Arthritis Medical Treatment and Home Care* (6th edition). Macmillan Company, New York, 1972.

BLAU, SHELDON PAUL, M.D. AND DODI SCHULTZ. *Arthritis: Complete, Up-to-Date Facts for Patients and Their Families*. Doubleday and Co., Inc., Garden City, New York., 1974.

BODANSKY, M. AND O. BODANSKY. *Biochemistry of Disease* (2nd edition). Macmillan Company, New York, 1952.

BONICA, JOHN J. *The Management of Pain*. Lea & Febiger, Philadelphia, 1954.

BRIDGES, M. A. *Dietetics for the Clinician*. Lea & Febiger, Philadelphia, 1936.

BROOKE, JAMES W. *Arthritis and You*. Harper, New York, 1960.

BRUCH, DR HILDE. *Eating Disorders: Obesity, and Anorexia Nervosa and the Person Within*. Basic Books, New York, 1973 and Routledge, London, 1973.

BURNETT, SIR MCFARLANE. *Natural History of Infectious Disease* (4th edition). Cambridge University Press, New York, 1972.

CALABRO, JOHN J., M.D. AND JOHN WYKERT. *The Truth About Arthritis Care*. David McKay Co., Inc., New York, 1971.

CLARK, STANLEY K., M.D., C.M., F.R.C.P. *What to Eat – and When* (9th edition). Pantagraph Press, Ltd., Bloomington, Ill., 1971.

COLLINS, W. DOUGLAS, M.D. *Illustrated Manual of Laboratory Diagnosis: Indications and Interpretations*. J. B. Lippincott Co., Philadelphia, 1968.

COOPER, F. L., et al. *Nutrition in Health and Disease* (14th edition). J. B. Lippincott Co., Philadelphia, 1958.

DAVIDSON, SIR STANLEY, A. P. MIKLEJOHN AND R. PASSMORE. *Human Nutrition and Dietetics*. Williams & Wilkins Co., Baltimore, 1959 and Churchill Livingstone, Edinburgh and London, 1972

DOWNING, JOHN GODWIN. *The Cutaneous Manifestations of Systemic Diseases*. Charles C. Thomas, Publisher, Springfield, Ill., 1954.

DUNBAR, ROBERT E. AND HOWARD F. SEGALL. *A Doctor Discusses Learning to Cope with Arthritis, Rheumatism, and Gout*. Budlong, Chicago, 1973.

ENGLE, GEORGE L. *Psychological Development in Health and Disease*. W. B. Saunders Co., Philadelphia, 1962.

EWART, CHARLES. *The Healing Needles: A Story of Acupuncture and Its Pioneer Practitioner, Dr. Louis Moss*. Elm Tree Books, Hamish Hamilton, London, 1972.

FIELD, HAZEL E. *Foods in Health and Disease*. Macmillan Company, New York, 1964.

FLATT, ADRIANEDE. *The Care of the Rheumatoid Hand*. Mosby, St Louis, 1974 and Kimpton, London, 1968.

FOOD AND NUTRITION BOARD. *Recommended Dietary Allowances* (7th edition). National Academy of Sciences, Washington, D.C., 1968.

FRIEDENWALD, J. AND J. RUHRA. *Diet in Health and Disease*. W. B. Saunders Co., Philadelphia, 1925.

GOFMAN, JOHN W., PH.D., M.D., ALEX V. NICHOLS, PH.D., AND

E. VIRGINIA DOBBIN. *Dietary Prevention and Treatment of Heart Disease.* G. P. Putnam's Sons, New York, 1958.

GOLDING, DOUGLAS M. *A Synopsis of Rheumatic Diseases* (2nd edition). Williams & Wilkins Co., Baltimore 1973 and Wright, Bristol, 1973.

GOOD, ROBERT A. AND DAVID W. FISHER (editors). *Immunobiology.* Sinauer Associates, Inc., Stamford, Conn., 1971

HARRIS, M. COLEMAN, M.D., AND NORMAN SHURE, M. D. *All About Allergy.* Prentice-Hall, Inc., Englewood Cliffs, N. J., 1969.

HAWKINS, HAROLD F. *Applied Nutrition.* Institute Press, Gardena, California., 1940.

HEYNINGEN, W. E. VAN. *Bacterial Toxins.* Charles C. Thomas, Publisher, Springfield, Ill., 1959.

HOLLANDER, JOSEPH LEE, M.D. *Arthritis and Allied Conditions: A Textbook of Rheumatology* (7th edition). Lea & Febiger, Philadelphia, 1956.

HORROBIN, DAVID F. *The Communication System of the Body.* Basic Books, New York, 1964.

HUEPER, W. C. AND W. D. CONWAY. *Chemical Carcinogenesis and Cancers.* Charles C. Thomas, Publisher, Springfield, Ill., 1965.

JAYSON, MALCOLM I. V., M.D., AND ALAN ST J. DIXON, M.D. *Understanding Arthritis and Rheumatism: A Complete Guide to the Problems and Treatment.* Pantheon Books, New York, 1974.

KEATS, ARTHUR S. *New Concepts in Pain and Its Clinical Management.* F. A. Davis Co., Philadelphia, 1967.

LAKESIDE LABORATORIES. *Metabolic Individuality and Diagnosis of Degenerative Disease.* Milwaukee, 1951.

LAMB, MINA W. AND MARGARETTE L. HARDEN. *The Meaning of Human Nutrition.* Pergamon Press, Inc., Elmsford, New York., 1973.

LEONARD, JON N., JACK L. HOFER AND NATHAN PRITIKIN. *Live Longer Now: The First One Hundred Years of Your Life: The 2100 Program.* Grosset & Dunlap, Inc., New York, 1974.

LEVI, LENNART (editor). *Society, Stress and Disease.* Vol. 1, *The Psychosocial Environment and Psychosomatic Diseases.* Oxford University Press, New York, 1971.

LEWIS, FAYE C. *All Out Against Arthritis.* Prentice-Hall, Inc., Englewood Cliffs, N.J., 1973.

LIEFMANN, DR ROBERT E. *Arthritis Discovery.* Commonwealth Publishing Co., Freeport, Bahamas, 1971.

McCARRISON, SIR ROBERT AND H. M. SINCLAIR. *Nutrition and Health.* Faber and Faber, London, 1953.

McCOLLUM, E. V. AND J. ERNESTINE BECKER. *Food, Nutrition, and Health* (3rd edition). Baltimore, 1934.

McCOLLUM, E. V. AND N. SIMMONDS. *The Newer Knowledge of Nutrition.* Macmillan Company, New York, 1929.

McDEVITT, HUGH O. AND MAURICE LANDY (editors). *Genetic Control of Immune Responsiveness.* Academic Press, London, 1972

McLESTER, J. S. *Nutrition and Diet in Health and Disease.* W. B. Saunders Co., Philadelphia, 1927.

MANN, FELIX, M.D. *Acupuncture: The Ancient Chinese Art of Healing and How It Works Scientifically.* Vintage Books, New York, 1971 and William Heinemann Medical Books Ltd., London, 1972

MANN, FELIX, M.D. *The Treatment of Disease by Acupuncture.* William Heinemann Medical Books Ltd., London, 1972.

*Medical Illustrations of Common Joint Diseases.* Eli Lilly & Co., Indianapolis, 1968.

MONIER-WILLIAMS, G. W. *Trace Elements in Food.* John Wiley & Sons, New York, 1949.

PAGE, IRVINE, M.D. *Speaking to the Doctor: His Responsibilities and Opportunities.* Proforum, Minneapolis, 1972.

PRICE, WESTON A. *Nutrition and Physical Degeneration.* American Academy of Applied Nutrition, Los Angeles, 1939.

QUIGLEY, D. T. *The National Malnutrition.* Lee Foundation for Nutritional Research, Milwaukee, 1943.

RAGEN, CHARLES AND ARTHUR I. SNYDER, *Rheumatoid Arthritis.* Yearbook Publishers, Chicago, 1955.

RAPAPORT, HOWARD G., M.D. AND SHIRLEY MOTTER LINDE, M.S. *The Complete Allergy Guide.* Simon & Schuster, Inc., New York, 1970.

RICHARDS, VICTOR. *Cancer: The Wayward Cell.* University of California Press, Berkeley, 1972.

ROSE, MARY SWARTZ. *The Foundations of Nutrition.* Macmillan Company, New York, 1933.

ROWE, ALBERT H., M.D. *Food Allergy.* Lea & Febiger, Philadelphia, 1931.

SHERMAN, H. C. *Chemistry of Food and Nutrition.* Macmillan Company, New York, 1932.

SCHMECK, HAROLD M. *Immunology: The Many-Edged Sword.* George Braziller, Inc., New York, 1974.

SMITH, RICHARD T. AND MAURICE LANDY (editors). *Immune Surveillance.* Academic Press, New York, 1970.

STERN, FRANCES. *Applied Dietetics*. Williams and Wilkins Co., Baltimore, 1943.

TAN, LEONG T., MARGARET Y.-C. TAN AND ILZA VEITH, M.D. *Acupuncture Therapy: Current Chinese Practice*. Temple University Press, Philadelphia, 1973.

TAUBE, E. LOUIS, M.D. *Food Allergy and the Allergic Patient: A Simple Review of Problems Encountered by the Recently Diagnosed Patient.* Charles C. Thomas, Publisher, Springfield, Illinois, 1973.

TURNER, JAMES S. (project director). *The Chemical Feast*. Ralph Nader Study Group Report on Food Protection and Food and Drug Administration, Grossman Publishers, Inc., New York, 1970.

WILLIAMS, ROGER, J. *Alcoholism: The Nutritional Approach*. University of Texas Press, Austin, 1959.

WILLIAMS, ROGER I. *Nutrition Against Disease: Environmental Prevention*. Pitman Publishing Co., New York, 1971.

WILLIAMS, SUE RODWELL. *Nutrition and Diet Therapy* (2nd edition). C. B. Mosby & Co., St. Louis, 1973.

WILSON, David. *Body and Antibody: A Report on the New Immunology*. Alfred A. Knopf Co., Inc., New York, 1971.

WINTON, ANDREW LINCOLN AND K. G. WINTON. *Structure and Composition of Foods* (2 volumes). John Wiley & Sons, 1935.

WOHL, M. G. AND R. S. GOODHART (editors). *Modern Nutrition in Health and Disease*. Lea & Febiger, Philadelphia, 1960.

WOLFF, HAROLD G. *Stress and Disease*. Charles C. Thomas, Publisher, Springfield, Ill., 1953.

WOLFF, STEWART AND HAROLD G. WOLFF. *Headaches: Their Nature and Treatment*. Little, Brown, Boston, 1953.

## Periodicals

AMMANN, ARTHUR J., M.D. 'How to Use Autoimmune Tests in Your Practice,' *Consultant*, March 1975, Vol. 15, No. 3, p. 55.

'Ankylosing Spondylitis Seems to Be Hereditary,' *JAMA*,* 19 August 1974, Vol. 229, No. 8, pp. 1035–6.

AREES, EDWARD A. AND JEAN MAYER. 'Monosodium Glutamate-Induced Brain Lesions: Electron Microscopic Examination,' *Science*, 30 October 1970, pp. 549–50.

'Arthritis and Drug Abuse,' *Medical Times*, September 1974, Vol. 102, No. 9, pp. 103–4.

* Journal of the American Medical Association.

AXLEROD, A. 'Nutrition in Relation to Acquired Immunity,' *Modern Nutrition in Health and Disease*, 1973.

BASKIND, MORTON S. 'The Technique of Nutritional Therapy,' *Journal of Applied Nutrition*, 1960, Vol. 13, No. 1.

BONICA, J. J., M.D. 'Acupuncture Anesthesia in the People's Republic of China,' *JAMA*, 2 September 1974, Vol. 229, No. 10, p. 1317.

BORTZ, E. L. 'Mechanisms of Aging,' *Journal of the American Geriatrics Society*, 1959, Vol. 7, p. 825.

BROOKS, CARTER D., M.D., et al. 'Tolerance and Pharmacology of Ibuprofen,' *Current Therapeutic Research*, April 1973, Vol. 15, No. 4, pp. 180–90.

BRYAN, WILLIAM J., JR., M.D., J.D., PH.D., L.L.D., F.A.I.H., F.A.C.M. 'The Law of Acupuncture,' *Journal of the American Institute of Hypnosis*, November 1973, Vol. 14, No. 6.

BUTTERWORTH, CHARLES E., JR., M.D. 'The Skeleton in the Hospital Closet,' *Nutrition Today*, March/April 1974.

CANNON, P. 'The Importance of Proteins in Resistance to Infection,' *JAMA*, 1945, Vol. 128, p. 360.

CLAUSEN, S. W. 'The Influence of Nutrition upon Resistance to Infection,' *Physiological Review*, 1934, Vol. 14, p. 309.

CROW, DR JAMES. 'Do Chemicals Sow the Seeds of Genetic Change?' *Medical World News*, 26 April 1968.

DALESSIO, D. J., M.D. 'Dietary Allergy in Vascular Headaches,' *JAMA*, 28 April 1975, Vol. 232, No. 4, p. 400.

'Dietary Fibre and Disease,' *JAMA*, 19 August 1974, Vol. 229, No. 8, p. 1068.

'Does Human Antibiotic Resistance Relate to Feed Supplements?' *Infectious Diseases*, December 1974, p. 3.

DOLE, V. P., et al. 'Dietary Treatment of Hypertension,' *Journal of Clinical Investigation*, 1951, Vol. 30, p. 1189.

EHRLICH, GEORGE E., M.D., 'Easing Pain Stiffness of Arthritis Outline,' *Chronic Disease*, October 1974.

FARRAR, J. T., M.D. 'There Is Too Much Stress On Bland Diet,' *Medical Opinion*, September 1974, pp. 31–6.

'Food Additives: Health Question Awaiting an Answer,' *Medical World News*, 7 September 1973, Vol. 14, No. 32, p. 72.

FRAZIER, CLAUDE E., M.D. 'Introduction to Allergy,' *Medical Insight*, June 1973, pp. 12–17.

'Gold Therapy in Rheumatoid Arthritis,' *Annals of Rheumatic Disease*, 1960, Vol. 19, p. 95.

'Gold Therapy in Rheumatoid Arthritis: Improving the Results,' *Consultant*, November 1974, pp. 95–7.

GOLDING, D. N., M.D., F.R.C.P.I. 'Problems in Rheumatology: Non-Articular Arthritis,' *Update International*, April 1974.

GOLDING, D. N., M.D. F.R.C.P.I. 'Variants in Rheumatology,' *Update International*, June 1974.

GRACE, LINDA. 'There Are No Harmless Substances,' *World Health*, April 1969, pp. 20–22.

HAGY AND SETTIPANE. 'Bronchial Asthma, Allergic Rhinitis and Alergy Skin Test Among College Students,' *Journal of Allergy*, December 1969, Vol. 44, No. 6.

HUANG, S., AND T. M. BAYLESS. 'Milk and Lactose Intolerance in Healthy Orientals,' *Science*, 1968, Vol. 160, pp. 83–4.

HURSH, L. M., M.D. 'Milk Has Something for Everybody?' *JAMA*, 5 May 1975, Vol. 232, No. 5.

JAMES, LYNNE, PH.D. 'Diet-Related Birth Defects,' *Nutrition Today*, July/August 1974, p. 4.

JOHNSON, PAUL E. 'Health Aspects of Food Additives,' *American Journal of Public Health*, June 1966, Vol. 56, No. 6.

'Joint Pain: Is It Really Rheumatoid Arthritis?' *Patient Care*, 1 May 1974, p. 27.

JUKES, THOMAS H., PH.D., D.SC. 'The Organic Food Myth,' *JAMA*, 14 October 1974, Vol. 230, No. 2, p. 276.

KEYS, A., et al. 'Lessons From Serum Cholesterol Studies In Japan, Hawaii and Los Angeles,' *Annals of Internal Medicine*, 1958, Vol. 48, pp. 83–94.

KHAIRI, M. RASHIDA, M.D., et al. 'Treatment of Paget Disease of the Bone (Osteitis Deformans): Results of a One-Year Study with Sodium Etidronate,' *JAMA*, 28 October 1974, Vol. 230, No. 4, pp. 562–7.

KLINGER, ALFRED D., M.D. 'Confronting Our Inadequate Nutrition,' *Medical Tribune*, 14 August 1974, p. 6.

LEVIN, MELVIN H., M.D. 'Gout: The Many Facets of Therapy,' *Consultant*, January 1974, pp. 27–9.

LITCHFIELD, JOHN T., JR., M.D. 'Drug Toxicity in the Human Fetus and Newborn,' *Applied Therapeutics*, September 1967, pp. 922–6.

LOONEY, GERALD L., M.D. 'Acupuncture Vindication May Lie in Basic Research,' *Modern Medicine*, April 1975, p. 128.

'Low Synovial Fluid Complement Linked to More Disabling Arthritis,' *Geriatrics*, March 1975, p. 193.

MACLAREN, WALTER R., M.D., F.A.C.A., et al. 'The Rat Masked Cell Degranulation Test As Applied to a Case of Severe Food Allergy,' *Annals of Allergy*, January 1972, Vol. 30, pp. 41–4.

'Major Breakthrough Against Arthritis,' *National Tattler*, 29 September 1974, Vol. 21, No. 13.

MALTZ, BERTRAM A., M.D. 'Guide to Arthritis Diagnosis,' *Chronic Disease*, May 1974.

MAYER, DR JEAN. 'What Every Doctor Should Know About Foods,' *Physician's World*, October 1974, Vol. 2, No. 10, p. 50.

MELNICK, ARNOLD, D.O. 'Helping the Child with Juvenile Rheumatoid Arthritis,' *Medical Opinion*, August 1974, p. 76.

MERKIN, CARL. 'Diet the Key to Controlling Arthritis,' *Prevention*, July 1974, pp. 134–43.

MICHELMORE, PETER. 'A Model Geriatric Health Care System: Coordinated Endeavour of Patient Care and Physician Training,' *Geriatrics*, February 1975, p. 146.

MORRISON, L. M., 'Diet in Coronary Arteroisclerosis,' *JAMA*, 1960, Vol. 173, pp. 884–8.

NELSON, JERE J., M.D. 'Relieving Select Symptoms of the Elderly,' *Geriatrics*, March 1975, Vol. 30, No. 3, p. 113.

'New Drugs May Soon Supplement Aspirin in Treating Arthritics,' *Medical News*, 29 July 1974, pp. 505–8.

'New Tests of Diet Urged as Coronary Disease Curb,' *Chronic Disease*, December 1974, Vol. 8, No. 12.

'The Nutrition Factor: Its Role in National Development,' *Nutrition Today*, November/December 1973, Vol. 8, No. 6.

'Nutritional Immunity: Host's Attempt to Withhold Iron from Microbial Invaders,' *JAMA*, 6 January 1975, Vol. 231, No. 1.

'Nutritional Immunity and Iron,' *Infectious Diseases*, December 1974, p. 9.

PERLMAN, HENRY HARRIS, M.D. 'The Formulary of Dermatologicals for Children,' *Drug Therapy*, January 1975, pp. 85–96.

PETERMAN, R. A. AND R. S. GOODHART. 'Current Status of Vitamin Therapy in Nervous and Mental Disease,' *Journal of Clinical Nutrition*, 1954, Vol. 2, pp. 11–21.

PRESS, EDWARD, M.D. AND LEONA YEAGER, M.D. 'Food Poisoning Due to Sodium Nicotinate,' *American Journal of Public Health*, October 1962.

RAPP, DORIS J., M.D. 'Milk Allergy from Birth to Old Age,' *Consultant*, September 1974, pp. 120–22.

'The Relationship to Brain Development and Behaviour,' *Nutrition Today*, July/August 1974, p. 12.

'Removing Artificial Colours, Flavours Reported Beneficial in MBD,' *Family Practice News*, Vol. 4, No. 13, p. 15.

RINZLER, S. H. 'Prevention of Heart Disease by Diet,' *Bulletin of the New York Academy of Medicine*, Vol. 44, pp. 936–49.

ROPES, M. W., et al. 'Proposed Diagnostic Criteria for Rheumatoid Arthritis,' *Bulletin of Rheumatic Diseases*, 1956, Vol. 7, p. 121.

RUDDY, SHAUN AND HARVEY R. COLTEN. 'Rheumatoid Arthritis: Biosynthesis of Complement Protein by Synovial Tissues,' *The New England Journal of Medicine*, 6 June 1974, Vol. 290, No. 23, pp. 1284–8.

RUDOLPH, CHARLES J., JR., PH.D. 'Immunology and Nutrition,' *Osteopathic Annals*, July 1974, pp. 45–50.

'Safe Use of Chemicals in Foods: Council Statement,' *JAMA*, 18 November 1961, Vol. 178, No. 7, p. 749.

SAMTER, MAX, M.D., AND RAY BEERS, JR., M.D. 'Intolerance to Aspirin: Clinical Studies and Consideration of Its Pathogenesis,' *Annals of Internal Medicine*, May 1968, Vol. 68, No. 5.

SANDERS, HOWARD J. 'Food Additives,' *Chemical and Engineering News*, 1966.

SILBERBERG, R. AND M. SILBERBERG. 'Skeletal Growth and Articular Changes in Mice Receiving High-Fat Diet,' *Americal Journal of Pathology*, 1950, Vol. 26, p. 113.

SKOSEY, JOHN L., M.D., PH.D. 'Rheumatoid Arthritis: Overlooked, Underestimated, and Confusing,' *Consultant*, July 1974, pp. 23–7.

TAO, GEORGE. 'Chinese Food Therapy: High Blood Pressure and You.' *China Medical Reporter*, March 1973, Vol. 1, No. 2.

'Treating Infectious Arthritis,' *Infectious Diseases*, June 1974, p. 12.

'The Truth About Adverse Drug Reaction Deaths,' *Viewpoint*, 1974, pp. 67–70.

TURPEINEN, et al. 'Diet and Coronary Events,' *Journal of the American Dietetics Association*, 1968, Vol. 52, pp. 209–13.

'Using Drugs in Elderly: Specialist Gives 7 Rules,' *Chronic Disease*, March 1974, Vol. 8, No. 3, p. 2.

VINK, J. DE M., M.D. CH.B. 'The Arthritis Patient and Family Practice,' *Continuing Education for the Family Physician*, Vol. 3, No. 1. pp. 2–31.

WATSON, GEORGE. 'Note on Nutrition in Mental Illness,' *Psychological Reports*, 1960, Vol. 6, No. 202.

WATSON, GEORGE, AND A. L. COMREY. 'Nutritional Replacement for Mental Illness,' *Journal of Psychology*, 1954, Vol. 38, pp. 251–64.

WEISS, HARVEY J., M.D. 'Aspirin: A Dangerous Drug?' *JAMA*, 26 August 1974, Vol. 229, No. 9.

'What Consumers Should Know About Food Additives,' F.D.A. Publication No. 10, June 1962.

'White Whale Holds Hope for Antibody Studies of Human Autoimmune Disease,' *Infectious Diseases*, June 1974, p. 17.

WICHER, KONRAD, ROBERT E. REISMAN, M.D. AND CARL E. ARBESMAN, M.D. 'Allergic Reaction to Penicillin Present in Milk,' *JAMA*, 1969, Vol. 208, No. 1, p. 143.

WITTIG, HEINZ J., M.D. 'Diet for Children with Food Allergies,' *Drug Therapy*, January 1975, pp. 129–41.

Also many publications of The Arthritis Foundation, the U.S. Department of Health, Education, and Welfare, and the National Institutes of Health.

# Index

# Index